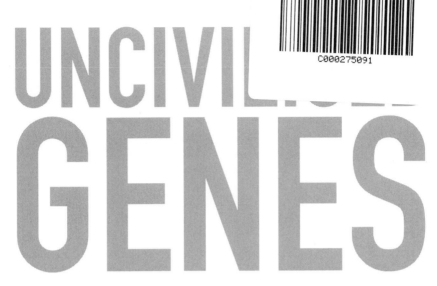

UNCIVILISED GENES

HUMAN EVOLUTION AND THE URBAN PARADOX

GUSTAV MILNE

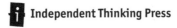

Independent Thinking Press

First published by

Independent Thinking Press
Crown Buildings, Bancyfelin, Carmarthen, Wales, SA33 5ND, UK
www.independentthinkingpress.com

Independent Thinking Press is an imprint of Crown House Publishing Ltd.

Cover images © Bastos and littleny – fotolia.com.
Author photograph © Andy Chopping/MOLA.

First published 2017.

A continuation of this page appears on page 264.

Edited by Ian Gilbert.

British Library Cataloguing-in-Publication Data
A catalogue entry for this book is available from the British Library.

Print ISBN 978-1-78135-265-6
Mobi ISBN 978-1-78135-282-3
ePub ISBN 978-1-78135-283-0
ePDF ISBN 978-1-78135-284-7

Printed and bound in the UK by
TJ International, Padstow, Cornwall

In commemoration of the life and work of
Dr Staffan Lindeberg (1950–2016)

Author of the pioneering study, *Food and Western Disease:
Health and Nutrition from an Evolutionary Perspective* (2010)

ACKNOWLEDGEMENTS

The origins of the Evolutionary Determinants of Health programme can be traced back to discussions with Professor Gordon Hillman and his students at University College London's Institute of Archaeology in the 1990s. Momentum gradually built thanks to the work, advice and support of Ben Gardner, Matt Pope, Professor Graham Rook, Ian Scott and Jemima Stockton at UCL, as well as Terrence Bettison (Living Streets). Following grants from the Ove Arup Foundation, UCL Grand Challenges and the UCL Transport Institute, a website was set up and a series of workshops were held, as well as the major conference in February 2014: Urban Paradox: Human Evolution and the 21st-Century Town. The work of Tom Cohen, Professor Stephen Marshall and Richard Tinnerman is duly acknowledged, as are the contributions to the conference and workshops from Nicola Christie, Abi Foster and Emma Karoune (and many others at UCL), as well as Bob Allies (Allies and Morrison Architects), Neil Davidson (J & L Gibbons), Lucy Saunders (Transport for London), Samir Singh (Arsenal in the Community) and Paola Spivach (Sustrans). Comments have also been gratefully received from anonymous reviewers, from many authors (see References and Further Reading), from Matt Morley (Biofit) and also from Professor Liz Pye, Professor Stephen Shennan and Professor Mark Thomas, together with Sonia Skaraas, Catherine Walker and especially from Charlotte Frearson, who also supplied many photographs for this volume. Last, but by no means least, the professionalism of Emma Tuck and the team at Crown House Publishing is most warmly acknowledged.

Nevertheless, in spite of their collective good works, the mistakes, misrepresentations or misunderstandings apparent in this book remain the sole responsibility of the author.

The book is dedicated to the cats with whom I have co-evolved and from whom I have learned much about the fluid boundaries between domestication and uncivilisation.

Gustav Milne
UCL Institute of Archaeology, London WC1H 0PY
Museum of London Archaeology,
46 Eagle Wharf Road, London N1 7ED

We gratefully acknowledge permission to publish material from the work of the following authors and publishers:

Wiley Global Permissions, for material taken from the late Dr Staffan Lindeberg's *Food and Western Disease* (2010) and B. Ridsdale's data used on pages 14–15: Comparing the causes of death in un-urbanised and urbanised communities, and again in Table 15.1: New world order.

Cambridge University Press and Professor R. Kelly for material taken from his 2013 study, 'The Lifeways of Hunter-Gatherers: The Foraging Spectrum', Table 3, p. 40 used in Appendix 1: Hunter-Gatherers with Latitude.

Professor L. Cordain for data used on page 80: Comparison of a hunter-gatherer style diet with a low-carbohydrate, a low-fat and a 'Mediterranean-type' diet, and on page 94: Working out.

M. Morley for his contribution (pages 111–112) Back to the gym?

Professor V. Harding and Professor D. Keene, for the map used on page 124: Parochial City.

Professor C. Roberts, for data used in Appendix 2: Diseases of Civilisation: Osteological Evidence from British Cemetery Excavations.

Professor R. Deaner for material used in Appendix 3: Hunting, Sport and a Gender Agenda.

CONTENTS

PROLOGUE

Telling tales

Once upon a time, in a land far, far away, was a beautiful country called Eden. And in this land was all the fresh water you could ever drink, all the fruit you could ever eat, all the creatures you could ever hunt and all the fish you could ever fish. The living was easy: the happy couple who lived there wanted for nothing. But, alas, it didn't last: Adam and Eve had to leave that beautiful garden and they, their children and their children's children had to work harder for a living in different, more hostile lands. That, at least, is how the ancient fable goes.

But modern science tells us that something similar did actually happen to the human race: we once lived in small tribes in wild, wide open spaces, walking, running, foraging and hunting, looking for food and water every day. We survived and procreated in tight tribal communities working with or fighting against natural forces that could as easily nurture us as destroy us. That's what our bodies and minds were designed to do, and that's exactly what we did for the first few million years of our ancient lives as 'hunter-gatherers'.

Uncivilised genes

But we have long left that Garden of Eden lifestyle, for today we live in towns with towering buildings, complex transport systems and high technologies. Modern urbanisation is a stunning development, a tribute to our remarkable resourcefulness, adaptability and great intelligence. But towns have only been around for less than 10,000 years, a very short time in the longer cycle of human evolution. By contrast, our ancestral hunter-gatherer regime sustained the human race for three million years or more – far longer than any other known civilisation or empire.

Beyond some relatively minor genetic variations, we have not, as yet, evolved anatomically to better accommodate to these new global urban conditions. Arguably, much of our mindset, emotions, instincts and intuitions are also largely unchanged. Subconsciously, a part of us believes we are still in Eden; physiologically we most certainly are. There is therefore a profound mismatch in the modern age between the urbanised world we are obliged to live in and the one we are genetically, metabolically, physiologically and psychologically better adapted for. Certainly most of us try to adapt culturally to town life: indeed, there are few other viable options. There has been a global expansion of urbanisation: cities are now the civilisation of the future. But

1

physiologically and psychologically, our genetic make-up remains much as it always was: uncivilised, un-urbanised and much misunderstood. That's not a derogatory comment about our Palaeolithic genome: it's just that urban life, in its present form, is not the environment we are genetically best adapted for. And just one of the direct consequences of this is the alarming rise in the prevalence of 'western lifestyle diseases' and conditions such as type 2 diabetes, sundry heart problems and rising obesity levels: it seems that towns are bad for us.

Building cities for humans

So how can we resolve this challenging conflict and make our own lives healthier and our urban lifestyles better? We cannot un-invent the 21st-century town, but by taking more notice of our Eden legacy, our ancient physiological and emotional roots, and by making good use of it on a daily basis, much could be improved. Various carrots, sticks, nudges and compromises that might be employed to effect such positive behavioural change are discussed in this book. If we could reshape our personal lives and the very fabric of our townscapes by basing the future on our shared past, then urban wellbeing will be significantly improved for all of us. We can't change our genes, but we can change our urban lifestyles to better fit our biology.

For the sake of our health and wellbeing, tomorrow's cities should be built for humans. And there is no time to delay, since by AD 2050, our global population will have risen from 7.2 billion to 9.6 billion (UN-DESA 2015). This book considers why and how we should be planning our modern towns and urban lifestyles, not so much for an uncertain future but on a proven prehistoric past. The better our cities are adapted to our uncivilised biology – the legacy of a lifestyle far older than urbanisation – the better we humans will adapt to them, and the healthier we will be. Our deep hunter-gatherer legacy – our Palaeolithic genome – still determines the quality of our health and much of how we instinctively think and respond, in spite of our new-found desire to be reasonable, logical and cost effective.

Chapter and verse

This book presents evidence-based research that suggests ways in which we can make a positive difference to modern life and town plans through developing and adopting more evolutionary-concordant behaviours and protocols. This book is *not* another celebrity-endorsed fad diet (although ancestral nutritional regimes are discussed in Chapters 4 and 5) and it is *not* another call to reject towns and seek solace in a rural idyll (although there is empathy with those who are so inclined). It is also *not* a rejection of modernity in favour of an imagined past – on the contrary, we are solidly situated deep within the 21st-century city – but it does offer suggestions as to how urban living might be reconfigured from a human evolutionary perspective.

Our ancient but largely uncivilised genes are introduced in Chapter 1. Culturally, society has changed at a remarkable speed, but anatomically and genetically we remain much as we were long before towns developed or even large-scale farming was adopted (Stringer and Andrews 2011, 236–239). There is consequently an aggressive mismatch between our Palaeolithic genome and the demands of modern urbanised living. Nevertheless, a better understanding of our deep past can materially benefit ourselves and our cities. In this chapter, we also ponder health, happiness and human nature from genetic as well as cultural viewpoints. The differences between the social and evolutionary determinants of health are then debated, insofar as they relate to the seemingly unstoppable increase in western lifestyle diseases. Remarkably, many of these conditions seem to have been rare or non-existent in non-urbanised communities enjoying evolutionary-concordant diets, as the detailed study of the Kitava islanders of Papua New Guinea has shown (Lindeberg 2010). There is thus a high price to pay for ignoring our uncivilised genes, since they seem to hold the key to good health and urban wellbeing.

The scientific archaeological evidence underpinning studies of our long-lived hunter-gatherer lifestyle is laid out in Chapter 2. The undirected evolution of our modern, omnivorous, two-legged upright physiology is plotted – a development that took six million years – and key aspects of the lifestyles of our ancient pre-agricultural, pre-urban ancestors are described. These may be profitably compared with another data set in Chapter 3, studies of non-urban tribal societies that survived into the modern era in environments as diverse as Australia, Africa, South America and the Arctic. These summary reviews of what we now call 'hunter-gatherer' regimes are based on ethnographic and anthropological research.

The next set of chapters detail the evolutionary determinants of health, by taking a particular hunter-gatherer theme, contrasting it with modern urban perspectives and finally offering possible resolutions to the challenges revealed by that mismatch. To open the discussion, Chapters 4, 5, 6 and 7 look at the evolutionary determinants of health and studies of the relatively well-rehearsed (if often misrepresented) nutrition and activity regimes. Moving on to less familiar ground, Chapters 8, 9 and 10 deal with the evolutionary determinants of social behaviour, while Chapters 11, 12, 13, 14 and 15 deal with urban wellbeing from a human evolutionary perspective.

We begin in Chapter 4 by considering archaeological evidence for Palaeolithic and Mesolithic diets as well as data from non-urbanised, hunter-gatherer societies that survived into the modern era. Chapter 5 reviews key common features of such regimes alongside modern 'western' diets and the diseases and conditions associated with them. Recent medical research is cited in support of the development of evolutionary-concordant nutritional regimes that better fit our unevolved digestive system.

Chapter 6 assesses the evolution of our ancient physiology and the physically active lifestyle of our ancestors. In Chapter 7 this is contrasted with the increasingly sedentary modern world, and suggestions are made for changing our lifestyle, buildings and town plans to better fit our bipedal physiology through the development of evolutionary-concordant activity regimes.

Attention turns to aspects of the hunter-gatherer mindset in Chapter 8, with a consideration of the psychology underpinning leadership and role models and the inclusive nature of ancient tribal societies. These often overlooked issues still resonate today in our huge, seemingly impersonal political conurbations and impact on the concepts of social hierarchy, community and neighbourhood, as well as social inclusion and exclusion.

Chapter 9 extends our study to the other aspects of modern life. For example, some forms of criminal activity, especially the urban gang, are shown to be an unwelcome perverse proxy for the hunting party. Evidence-based research is presented to show how some of its problems can be addressed head on through sport – for example, as in the Midnight Basketball project in the United States and the Kickz football programme in the UK. Both of these are positive, evolutionary-concordant approaches to such antisocial behaviour.

In Chapter 10 we consider how ancient societies communicated through body language, and particularly through rhythm and music, for identity, for emotion, for celebration and for memory. One of the evolutionary determinants of music – the evolution of the human voice box – can be shown to be earlier than the development of spoken language. Music is part of our resilient preliterate hunter-gatherer legacy, a welcome attribute of urban wellbeing in the computer age.

Hunter-gatherers lived in wild, wide open spaces, superficially the very antithesis of a modern town. However, our essential biophilia, the direct connection with 'nature', need not and should not be severed from city life, as research in Chapter 11 reports. A detailed discussion of the role and value of urban greenspace in its many forms is presented, viewed not just as passive one-dimensional landscaping but from deeper physiological and psychological viewpoints. Crucially, microbiological research by Professor Graham Rook and his team is summarised in Chapter 12 – work which has revolutionised our understanding of the active relationship in our physical engagement with the natural world. This concerns the microbiota we have co-evolved with as well as the workings (or, increasing today, the failings) of our immune system. This paradigm-shifting work shows that parks and pets are just as important to our continuing good health as evolutionary-concordant diet and exercise regimes.

Taking the lessons learned thus far, the next chapters also break new ground, taking a summary look at town planning and urban wellbeing from a human evolutionary perspective. Chapter 13 considers how urban settlements have developed over the centuries from a public health standpoint, with the work of the Roman architect Vitruvius through to Sir Ebenezer Howard's garden cities, New Urbanism and the Healthy Cities movement.

This leads directly to Chapter 14. Here we can do no more than open a discussion on how modern town planning can effectively build on evolutionary-concordant principles to maximise urban wellbeing in the design of tomorrow's cities. The necessary impetus for this study is that a rising population of an extra three billion souls will have to be housed in new towns across the globe within the next 30 years. Among the many issues that must be addressed is the need for cleaner urban air, since our Palaeolithic respiratory systems still cannot cope with toxic fumes and diesel particulates. Some consideration is also given to modern residential buildings, on the importance of windows and rooms with a view, and on how office, schools and hospitals can be designed to be more evolutionary concordant, and thus more effective institutions.

In conclusion, Chapter 15 considers how we, although biologically still broadly Palaeolithic, can nevertheless adapt more successfully to an urbanised modern world. A series of guidelines, the 'Eden Protocol', are suggested, covering personal and institutional health behaviours as well as templates for building design and town planning. Here, the term 'Eden' is used as an abbreviation for the evolutionary determinants of health and urban wellbeing, while 'Protocol' is used to describe a series of suggested procedures designed to encourage evolutionary-concordant behaviour; they are just that, suggestions to open a new debate, and are not directives, regulations or statutes of the realm. Nevertheless, through the development and adoption of such protocols we might make a difference to 21st-century life by adopting ones that are more in tune with our basic physiology, psychology, metabolism and mindset.

This book therefore promotes the concept that human evolutionary con-cordance is the unifying paradigm underpinning not just personal wellbeing, but also institutional wellbeing and urban wellbeing. Our ancient and unciv-ilised genes have a real role to play in planning our modern urban futures. But to get there, we need some archaeology, anthropology, microbiology, neuroscience, evolutionary genetics, philosophy, nutritional science, psychol-ogy, crime science and common sense. And also an understanding of pets, architecture, town planning, gardening, football, shopping, picnics, bicycles, the sound of music and why there's nothing like an open fire.

Chapter 1

IN THE BEGINNING

This strange message Darwin brings,

… apes and men,

Blood-brethren.

Thomas Hardy (1840–1928)

Irreconcilable differences

What did the Romans ever do for us? One of their great cultural and social contributions was towns: they introduced us to the civilising concept of urbanisation. However, that came at a price, since study of their cemeteries in Britain shows that they also provided the first evidence in these islands for scurvy, rickets, osteomalacia, Reiter's syndrome, gout, ankylosing spondylitis, rheumatoid arthritis, psoriatic arthritis, septic arthritis, tuberculosis, osteitis, poliomyelitis and leprosy. None of these diseases or conditions were seen in the prehistoric, largely un-urbanised tribal populations that lived here before the Roman invasion of AD 43. So civilisation seems to have been a mixed blessing.

Today, most of us live in towns, but are modern cities any better for us? There is, unfortunately, clear evidence from the ever growing list of 'western lifestyle diseases' – the alarming increase in obesity, type 2 diabetes and cardiovascular problems to name but a few – that urban life even in the 21st century can actually be bad for our wellbeing. One of the key reasons is that so much of our current urban culture is not concordant with our ancient but largely unchanged basic biology. This evolved over many millennia to support a quite different lifestyle in a quite different environment. This book discusses that seemingly irreconcilable mismatch between modern urban living and our uncivilised genes but, in conclusion, it suggests solutions to this very real challenge.

For most of the long period of human evolution, a period of up to six million years, our race and their direct ancestors lived off the land and not in towns. We humans once shared a common ape-like ancestor with the chimpanzee. But some time between four and seven million years ago those two distinct lineages diverged. After that, over some 300,000 generations, the unique attributes of our human physical form gradually developed, including our upright posture and a larger brain size, as we entered the Old Stone

Age or Palaeolithic period (see e.g. Itan et al. 2010). For most of this time, we were foragers or hunter-gatherers, living off the land in small tribal societies, developing a working (if not always harmonious) relationship with nature. A particular part of our genetic make-up evolved over this long era to support that lifestyle. We have all inherited a complete set of those genes, a bundle of genetic material still encoded in our modern DNA, called here our 'Palaeolithic genome'.

The most significant cultural changes in this long period occurred just some 5,000 to 10,000 years ago, the period often called the Neolithic Revolution. This saw the development of widespread agriculture (large-scale plant and animal husbandry) and then, reliant upon the considerable surpluses produced, the establishment of towns, cities, states and empires. These new developments had a profound impact on all aspects of society, including its organisation and the ownership, acquisition and defence of land and territories. There was also a detrimental effect on human nutrition and health, evident in the bones of those early farmers and town dwellers, and still largely unresolved today. The physiology that had slowly evolved over some 300,000 generations to effectively husband and process the products of a daily hunting and gathering regime has only had about 300 generations to accommodate to the radically new world order. The marked contrast between the breakneck speed with which our urbanised culture is now developing and the glacial pace with which our biology responds to the new demands is producing huge pressure on our wellbeing.

Human nature?

What makes us do what we do, and why do we do it? There are at least four agents involved here: our genetic make-up, our genetic mindset, our culture and our reason. It is hard to estimate which is the greater driver of our daily lives. All four have a significant part to play, although their precedence will vary with time or circumstance. While both the latter two can and do alter each other, both are heavily influenced by the immutable force of the first pair, our genes.

To start with, our genetic make-up and mindset – that is, the physical and behavioural inheritance of our Palaeolithic genome. This dictates not just the colour of our eyes, hair, skin and such 'natural' talents as we may possess – features which vary from family to family – but also a common set of innate, instinctive, basic emotional responses, developed during the long evolutionary period when humans and their immediate ancestors were foragers. The instincts and attributes of our genetic behaviour were developed to facilitate survival and procreation in an uncertain world. They encompass our need for survival, for society, for fight or flight, a capacity for violence, a capacity for love. Many of them could be considered under the commonly heard phrase 'human nature', but arguably might be better termed 'primate nature', since the origins of such attributes are rather older than humanity. They are acquired from our parents, who acquired them from their parents, ad infinitum, and that same genetically coded bundle will likewise be passed on to our children. Some strong emotions and drives are included in this package, still reflecting those survival instincts embedded in our deep past. They are neither right nor wrong, but in today's very different urban environment, some must be redirected by a moral or cultural compass.

This leads us to the next key influence on our lives, the culture we grew up in. This encompasses the family values we absorbed as children, whatever schooling we had, the social mores, customs, work ethic and lifestyles observed around us, together with the contemporary laws and religion, lapsed or otherwise. These influences are not imposed on a 'blank slate' of a mind, but on top of the instincts, intuition and emotional responses we were born with. All these cultural elements are thus not innate, but acquired part-consciously, part-unconsciously, during our lifetime. As such, they cannot be transmitted to the next generation through our genes, but they can still be passed on to our children, or indeed anybody else (depending on how receptive they choose to be), through education and through the almost universal ability of humans to imitate each other.

The biologist Richard Dawkins, however, has suggested that each concept we learn or adopt could, in the same way as genes, evolve in its own right as it is itself passed on and then replicated by its new host (Dawkins 1976). These units of culture have been termed 'memes', although there is still discussion about the precise definition. That ideas change as they are passed from person to person or from generation to generation is indisputable, but similarities with our current understanding of genetic development is arguably figurative.

Whatever the actual process of cultural transmission might be, it's clear that humans are social animals: living in herds and learning to ape what your successful neighbour does can have evolutionary advantages. But living together in large herds also requires traffic lights to avoid too many collisions, and thus city life needs the imposition of ground rules and regulations upon which such an ever-changing urban culture can evolve. And that brings us to our fourth and final factor, our reason – the human ability to think logically and widely, arguably the one and only measure that separates us from (most of) the animal kingdom. Our ability to think through scientific questions has enabled us to develop the technologies we depend upon, but daily take for granted: we invented the mathematics upon which it is all predicated. We also developed the languages that transmit information at all levels, from the mundane to the highly complex. In the multimedia world we inhabit today, we have ready access to information and ideas on an unprecedented scale.

For much of our daily life there may be little overt conflict between nature and nurture, between our genes and our culture: indeed there is considerable crossover. However, there are situations in which nature may pull in one direction, nurture in another. In theory, we should be able to use our superior brain power to moderate between the two, defining a prudent, socially acceptable, legally correct and morally defensible course of action. But do we? If we did, then brutal wars would never get started. Even at the most mundane level, given a choice of menu, do we select the most nutritious meal, the most attractive, the cheapest or the sweetest? In our 21st-century world, which speaks loudest: our reason, our culture or our Palaeolithic genome?

Genetically speaking, 'happiness' is best seen as part of nature's reward system, an endorphin-charged response to an activity or situation that our Palaeolithic genome regards as good for our survival: eating, socialising, mating and so forth. Alas, it is a system designed for a half-remembered past to sit beside other deep responses, such as fight or flight, survival instincts for an uncertain and unreasonable world. Today, overeating can still elicit the same psychological feel-good feeling in your mind during the meal itself, but this will subsequently be tempered by your Palaeolithic physiology's response to material it cannot sensibly digest.

It is therefore all too possible that our "cultural-inheritance system can run counter to the genetic one", if we develop a lifestyle that is "maladaptive from the biological reproductive success point of view" (Shennan 2003, 19) – that is to say, one that is bad for us from an evolutionary perspective. It is the central assertion of this book that many aspects of our currently evolving urban lifestyles are doing just that: running counter to the demands of our Palaeolithic genome and consequently offering no evolutionary advantages. This mismatch of genetics and culture can be resolved, however, as this book tries to show.

Urban wellbeing: social and evolutionary determinants of health

Complex social, cultural, political and economic factors all contribute to health or ill health in our modern urban societies. As Professor Sir Michael Marmot's social determinants of health initiatives have demonstrated, good health and enhanced wellbeing tends to improve with social class (Rydin et al. 2012, 1). Those living in the most deprived areas of a city such as Glasgow, for example, have a life expectancy that is 12 years shorter than their neighbours in more affluent districts. Addressing the social inequalities of health that people are born into remains a major concern, and still requires political, economic and cultural change (Marmot and Wilkinson 2006, 1).

It is not, however, just differing socio-economic status that leads to poor health. This was shown 60 years ago in a landmark study of London buses (or, rather, their crew) at a time long before one-person operated vehicles were the norm. In 1953, the bus driver would sit isolated and imprisoned in his cab all day. The conductor, by contrast, would move around the bus, up and down the stairs, working the upper deck as well as the lower, interacting with the passengers. For the purposes of the study, the drivers and conductors were all male, were all from the same social class and all worked the same routes. But there were alarming differences in their health profiles, with a significantly higher mortality rate and susceptibility to coronary heart disease among the drivers than the conductors. For example, the immediate mortality rate following a heart attack was twice as high for drivers as for conductors (Morris et al. 1953a, 1953b). Similar studies have been conducted in other countries at other dates but, alas, with similar results (Tse et al. 2006). Regardless of social class, daily exercise (or lack of it) is a key evolutionary determinant of health.

Our concern in this book is therefore with that more fundamental mismatch which exists between our Palaeolithic genome and modern urban living, between the artificially modified Anthropocene world we currently live in (Zalasiewicz et al. 2010; see also 'Brave new epoch', page 12) and the environments we are genetically, metabolically, physiologically and psychologically best adapted for (see e.g. Coward et al. 2015). It is on these related issues that the evolutionary determinants of health programme focuses: facing up to the challenge presented by the alarming rise in western lifestyle diseases and other associated problems. Unlike the social determinants of health, the immutable evolutionary determinants of health that we are all born with – such as the prime need for daily exercise – cannot be changed. It is our towns and urban lifestyles that must be changed instead.

Brave new epoch

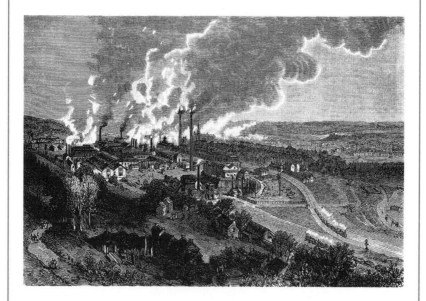

Satanic mills: the Industrial Revolution in the 18th century not only transformed society, but also began irreversible changes to the global environment.

Scientists studying the deep past have divided the earth's development into broad eras, subdivided into geological periods, then epochs, then ages, all based on identifiable and significant observable changes in, for example, rock formations, glacial advances, global changes in temperature and sea levels. We humans are living at the very end of the Quaternary period: our direct ancestry can be traced back into the Miocene epoch (over 20 million years ago), through various ice ages into the Pliocene (c. 3.5 million years ago) and Pleistocene (2.5–1.25 million years ago) and then into the Holocene.

But recent research suggests that we are now entering a new epoch called the Anthropocene. Unlike the previous stages in the earth's development, this time period is not defined by the natural forces and cycles of nature, but by the interference of humans in those cycles. A list of broadly simultaneous global 'markers' can be traced, such as increases in the fallout of particulates from burning fossil fuels and the substantial modification of carbon, nitrogen and phosphorus cycles; widespread changes in vegetation and accelerating rates of extinction of animal species; rates of sea-level rise and the extent of human influence in the climate system, all significantly exceeding changes noted in the Late Holocene. The future does not look good: indeed a Doomsday scenario, variously termed the Anthropocene, Holocene or Sixth Extinction, has been proposed (Kolbert 2014).

Arguably, the origins of these profound developments might be traced back to the Neolithic period, which saw the beginnings of the movement towards greater population density, clearance of forests for agriculture and transformation of soils for cropping, not to mention the conscious selection of plants for intensive cultivation and animals for breeding stock (Fuller et al. 2015). That said, the developments associated with the increased urbanisation and the 18th-century Industrial Revolution most certainly made their indelible mark. The march of our urbanised civilisations has indeed changed the world, but not quite in the way that was once envisaged. To survive in this new epoch, humanity must now learn to better adapt, not just to urban life but to a changing world of its own making.

An urban advantage?

The so-called 'urban advantage' – the assumption that those living in towns have greater health benefits than their rural neighbours – should not be considered as a foregone conclusion: not only do "rich and poor still live in different epidemiological worlds even in the same city" (Rydin et al. 2012, 1), but different aspects of living (e.g. diet) might be demonstrably more 'healthy' in the country than in modern towns. Indeed, for the new urban populations in expanding 18th- and 19th-century western conurbations, outcomes such as average age at death or levels of infant mortality actually *increased* before sanitary conditions began improving in the later decades of that period. In theory, as income per capita rises, so too should life expectancy, based on a steady reduction in death rates as well as higher birth rates. But the global picture is rather more complex. Although stringent public health measures and much improved health services removed many of the initial scourges of city life, such as cholera and typhoid, those evils seem to have been replaced by an increasing catalogue of diseases and conditions whose presence and profile were far less significant in the previous era. Many of these new villains are a direct product of our current urban lifestyles – that is, they are largely part of a culture of our own making.

Support for such an assertion comes from the work of Dr Staffan Lindeberg and his detailed study of the population of Kitava, an unmodernised community on an isolated island in Papua New Guinea. The causes of death there seem to have excluded diseases and conditions such as coronary and stroke-related conditions, atherosclerosis, type 2 diabetes, obesity, insulin resistance, high blood pressure, dyslipidaemia, dementia, breast, colorectal and prostate cancer, osteoporosis, rickets and autoimmune diseases such as multiple sclerosis. It is accepted that we all have to die from some cause some day. Nevertheless, it is surely significant that, according to figures from the World Health Organization (WHO 2004), 52.1% of the most modern, urbanised global population died of conditions or diseases that were rare or non-existent in the non-urbanised population from Kitava (see box 'Death in the city'). Arguably a case could be made for a non-urban advantage.

Death in the city

Table 1.1. Comparing the causes of death in un-urbanised and urbanised communities

	Non-urbanised	Urbanising	Urbanised	Highly urbanised
Accidents/homicide	Y			
Neonatal infections	Y	8		
Malarial infections etc.	Y	9		
Prematurity/low birth weight	Y	10		
Diarrhoeal disease	N	3		
HIV	N	4		
Tuberculosis	N	7	10	
Road traffic accidents	N		6	
Hypertensive heart disease	N		7	
Coronary heart disease	N	2	2	1
Stroke/cerebrovascular disease	N	5	1	2
Trachea/bronchus/lung cancer	N		5	3
Lower respiratory infections	N	1	4	4

	Non-urbanised	Urbanising	Urbanised	Highly urbanised
Chronic obstructive pulmonary disease	N	6	3	5
Alzheimer's/dementia	N			6
Colon/rectum cancers	N			7
Diabetes	N		9	8
Breast cancer	N			9
Stomach cancer	N		8	10

Source: Lindeberg 2010; Ridsdale and Gallop 2010, 4.1.

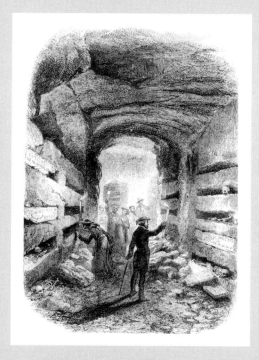

Resting in peace? Urban dead interred in catacombs.

Table 1.1 lists the most common causes of death in different communities across the world. Column 1 is based on results of a population study of a non-urban ancestral nutrition and activity regime (Y = common; N = rare or non-existent) from Kitava, in Papua New Guinea, which is compared with detailed data from the 2004 World Health Organization global survey of low-, middle- and high-income urban populations. The ranking (1–10) represents the most common cause of death (1) to the tenth most common cause of death (10) in that group. Note that the prime causes of death change as global populations become more urbanised (columns 2–4).

Column 1 presents the picture for an un-urbanised community living a hunter-gatherer type lifestyle that very broadly represents how humans may have survived for some three million years. It should be stressed that there is (or was) an immense variety of communities living in widely differing environments, all pursuing differing versions of what could be loosely termed 'hunter-gathering' (Kelly 2013). The data for the example presented here were collected in the Trobriand Islands, which support a population of 23,000 people, and where Dr Lindeberg led a long-term research project on the island of Kitava. The communities there had active lifestyles and nutritional regimes incorporating fish, fruit, roots and other vegetables, and 6% of the population lived to between 60 and 95 years of age.

The data from that un-urbanised society are compared with the ranking of the ten most common causes of death recorded in societies across the globe which are urbanising (columns 2 and 3) or fully urbanised (column 4). The last three columns could therefore serve as a proxy for the process of urbanisation itself and its impact on the health of the population.

Data in these three columns were collated for the World Health Organization in 2004 (broadly contemporary with the Kitava study) and list the then ten most common causes of death in contemporary low-, medium- and high-income countries. Here these categories are taken as proxies for cultures that are urbanising, urbanised and highly urbanised.

There is a clear relationship between three of the most common causes of death noted in Kitava (column 1) and in the low-income urbanising population (column 2), with issues such as infant mortality and malaria. That these are preventable or containable is demonstrated by their non-appearance in the top ten causes listed for middle- and high-income populations (columns 3 and 4 respectively).

The table shows that modern treatments have indeed had an effective impact on major problems associated with, for example, childbirth, malaria and tuberculosis. The latter is first listed in column 2, but does not appear in the top ten most common causes of death in high-income countries, representing progress on the public health front. However, new urban issues are introduced in columns 2 and 3, such as road traffic accidents, diabetes, cancers and coronary heart disease.

For the high-income, most urbanised societies represented in column 4, neither road traffic accidents nor any of the other eight conditions listed at the head of the table figure in the top ten most common causes of death. This represents genuine benefits from effectively regulated urbanisation. That said, the new entrants in column 4 include Alzheimer's and various cancers, while diabetes rises to eighth place and lung cancer to third. Taking all cancers together, they comprise 13% of the total, but coronary heart and stroke-related diseases still remain above 25% of the total.

So why is it that the ten most common causes of death in modern, highly urbanised populations (column 4) were rare or non-existent in un-urbanised Kitava (column 1)?

Reverse approach

Setting aside relocating to Papua New Guinea, what can be done to make our modern urban lifestyles more in line with the health profiles of the Kitava population? Modern medical research is often reactive, and tends to target specific diseases, their potential triggers or the effects and impacts of potential pharmaceutical remedies for particular conditions. It must be stressed that major benefits have resulted from this highly focused approach to the molecular and physiological mechanisms underlying what is termed the proximate mechanical cause of a particular condition.

Our project, however, takes a different perspective, looking at the major challenge presented by western lifestyle diseases – the so-called 'diseases of affluence'. Given that a substantial part of our genetic make-up (our Palaeolithic genome) is basically the same for the Kitava population, it follows that the profound difference in the most common causes of death between them must reflect significant differences in diet, activities and/or environment. It seems that the more urbanised we become, the more susceptible we are to adverse conditions of our own making. So, instead of considering why and how modern city dwellers contract coronary heart disease, the reverse approach is adopted here: the question we should be asking is why the Kitava population do *not* suffer from that or any of the cancers and other conditions that are now all too common in the West. Rather than mounting attacks on these conditions individually, this reverse approach enables all these diseases to be considered as a group: sick city syndrome. Faster and more effective progress might be made if the root cause of the syndrome is addressed upstream at source, rather than waiting for major flood events downstream.

Eden Protocol

We need to reconfigure our diet and activity regimes as well as our social and urban environment so that our Palaeolithic genome is persuaded into operating 'as normal', rather than continuing to endure the (literally) abnormal and unnatural demands made upon it that have such devastating consequences for our health. Once the effective 'healthy' differences between an ancestral lifestyle and a modern urban lifestyle have been identified, then work can begin on devising possible solutions. Proxy behaviours and simulated environments can then be introduced to our 21st-century towns, allowing us to enjoy the benefits of urbanisation while reversing such evils as the rising obesity epidemic with all its many associated problems.

The first stage is the identification of key positive physiological and psychological components of an ancestral lifestyle, regarding nutrition, activity, societal issues and engagement with nature (essential for an effective immune system). Next comes the formulation of evolutionary-concordant protocols that can be readily adopted in a 21st-century context, as well as in urban design guidelines. A combination of personal and institutional health behaviours (called Eden Protocols in this book) coupled with more evolutionary-concordant public health programmes are therefore suggested, extending current initiatives and relevant research already in the public domain. The lessons of human evolutionary archaeology could thus become central to the reconfiguration of urban lifestyles and planning for the next generation of cities.

The meaning of life

Adopting these evolutionary-concordant protocols should lead to improved urban wellbeing, but what precisely is meant by that rather overused term 'wellbeing'? 'Life, liberty and the pursuit of happiness' is a familiar phrase, and a worthy sentiment to underpin society in the modern age. The first two pillars, life and liberty, are more or less straightforward, but the third is easier to recognise than define (e.g. Layard 2005). Hedonists see happiness simply as pleasure and the absence of pain for the individual, while others – from Aristotle onwards – argue that wellbeing (eudaimonia) should define a good and virtuous life, one that contributes to a happier society. All the sovereign states recognised by the United Nations subscribe to its System of National Accounts, which includes the measure of gross domestic product (GDP) as the primary indicator of economic production within a country through the calculation of income, whether by individuals, businesses or government. This figure does not, however, take into account a number of major social, health and environmental issues (e.g. employment rates, infant mortality, longevity), and thus there is no obvious relationship between rising GDP and the rising contentment of the population (Stiglitz et al. 2010).

The distinguished economist Professor Richard Layard discussed these issues in his influential 2005 study, before posing a question. Although a modern, urbanised, technologically pioneering economy can increase its GDP year on year, could it simultaneously increase the general wellbeing of its people? For those living in abject poverty, or indeed in relative poverty, the answer is obviously yes: nobody wants to be hungry, homeless, destitute or desperate. There is no doubt that, for those who currently see themselves as 'poor', our economy and society can provide the money to buy a way out of material poverty. But once an acceptable standard of living has been achieved, what then? Professor Layard demonstrates that, although the material wealth and average income of the population in Britain and the United States over the last 50 years has significantly increased, the 'happiness' of the population has not. There is, in fact, evidence of a reverse trend: instances of depression and mental health problems are apparently on the increase in these materially 'better-off' societies. This all too clearly confirms the Easterlin paradox, named after the eponymous professor of economics at the University of Southern California (Easterlin 1974). In answer to the question, 'Does economic growth improve the human lot?', evidence was presented to show that, contrary to expectation, happiness at a national level does not increase with wealth once basic needs are fulfilled. As an example, the measure of the Fordham Index of Social Health (FISH) has actually deteriorated in the United States since 1973, even though GDP has increased. The FISH index measures 16 socio-economic factors, including rates of infant mortality, poverty among the elderly and unemployment, as well as housing and income inequality.

Defining moment

However it is measured, there is now a general consensus that the mainte-nance and promotion of physical and psychological wellbeing for the entire population is a precondition of a more prosperous and cohesive society. For the purposes of this book, a basic question must therefore be asked and answered: what do we mean by 'good health' and 'wellbeing', or indeed by their contrary states 'ill health' and 'ill-being'? Peace was once famously described as the absence of war, based on the assumption that neither of those two elements represented normality: life was ever in flux, moving inexorably from one to the other. Should good health and ill health be seen in the same light, each being defined solely as the absence of the other? Or should we take a more positive, proactive line and suggest that good health be considered as the expected norm and ill health the abnormal state?

The constitution of the World Health Organization, as adopted in New York in June 1946, defined health not just as the absence of disease or infirmity, but as a state of complete physical, mental and social wellbeing. In 2008, the New Economics Foundation added that wellbeing should also include how people feel and function (Abdallah et al. 2008, 7–8). For this book, those definitions are carried forward and expanded.

Our basic physiology, metabolism and mindset are all determined by our long human evolution. This shows us what we were (and still are) genetically designed to do, and, conversely, but just as crucially, what we were not designed to do. We were designed, for example, to eat fresh food and take daily exercise. Our overburdened National Health Service is all too well aware of the complications that arise from an urban population that ignores these fundamental evolutionary determinants of health, as the incidence of obesity, diabetes, cardiovascular problems and several forms of cancer all too painfully prove. As Professor Marmot eloquently states, "Although our material and social environments have changed beyond recognition over the last 10,000 years … our underlying biology is essentially the same as it was in ancient Babylon" (Brunner and Marmot 2006, 13). Archaeologists heartily agree with his sentiment, but would respectfully add many millennia to his chronology.

Here, wellbeing and good health (physical and mental) are defined as the product of following evolutionary-concordant behaviours. Ill health is partially the converse, a lifestyle that deviates from that broad path and is impacted by the associated consequences, or one that is affected by infectious or contagious diseases, a common occurrence in conurbations. Guidance for a healthy lifestyle, reflecting and respecting the legacy of human evolution, is summarised in the protocols suggested in Chapter 15.

In summary, *normality* in health terms is working with our Palaeolithic genome; poor health is therefore abnormal, too often the product of a lifestyle that is not evolutionary concordant. *Good health* is the consequence of adopting evolutionary-concordant behaviour – for example, the proxy nutritional regimes, societal systems and lifestyle-embedded activities that all correspond to and are required by that concept. *Urban wellbeing* is a state of mind and body obtained by those who have adopted evolutionary-concordant behaviours within an urban environment modified on evolutionary-concordant lines.

Measuring your happiness

The simple, mechanistic measurement of a nation's GDP is currently no longer considered the only guide to developmental progress. Since "people are the real wealth of a nation", as a 1990 United Nations Human Development Report stated, the focus of our attention has now shifted to increasing human wellbeing, as much as economic growth. The United Nations Human Development Index (HDI) is therefore based on the assumption that economic growth will not necessarily equate to increased wellbeing, and thus sets out to measure the positive or negative impact of such development on people's health, education and income. The ratings range from the highest score of 1.000 right down to 0.000. The HDI measures such attributes as GDP per person, equitable distribution of income, access to education and adult literacy, years of schooling and life expectancy, as well as achievements in health and gender equity.

Measuring happiness is not without its challenges. It has been argued that there is increasing confusion and blurring of the concepts of 'happiness', 'contentment', 'wellbeing' (economic, social or personal) and 'good health'. Exactly what is being quantified, and how that is achieved, depends initially on precisely why such a survey is required: children, adults, senior citizens, farmers, fishermen and the very rich all have different perspectives. Should the basic unit be an individual, a household or a state? What is more revealing, a macro- or a micro-analysis? We now have a rather confusing number of guides: there is a Genuine Progress Indicator, an Index of Sustainable Economic Welfare, Gallup regularly polls 130 nations to ascertain global happiness, Bhutan has developed the concept of Gross National Happiness and the World Health Organization has a Quality of Life Index.

France recently commissioned a major report on wellbeing with its 12 detailed recommendations to audit the national *joie de vivre* (OECD 2013), and the UK, through the Office for National Statistics, has been reporting its own annual survey of national wellbeing since 2012. These reports include studies relating wellbeing to 'health', 'where we live', 'household and families' and 'what we do' (ONS 2012). Similar strategies have now been adopted by Wales and Denmark, for example. The definition, development and measurement of human wellbeing are all now centre stage: our happiness is no longer just our concern, or an issue for philosophic or hedonistic debate, but is a matter for governmental enquiry.

Chapter 2

GENESIS

… with all his noble qualities … with his god-like intellect which has penetrated into the movement and constitution of the solar system – with all these exalted powers – Man still bears in his bodily frame the indelible stamp of his lowly origins.

Charles Darwin (1809–1882)

A garden in Eden

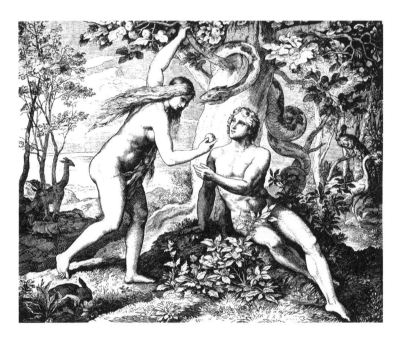

Figure 2.1. A Garden in Eden: the mythical first hunter-gatherers enjoy the fruits of the field.

All cultures have their creation myths, their tales of how life began: the Book of Genesis, the first book in the Old Testament, records just such a tale. Translated by Tyndale from Greek and ancient Hebrew in the 16th century, the fable of the six-day wonder is familiar throughout the western world, but rather more for its ringing, poetic prose than its scientific content. "In the beginning," we are told, "God created the heavens and the earth. And the earth was without form, and void; and darkness was upon the face of the deep ... And God said, Let there be light: and there was light."

As well as day and night, land and sea, and all manner of plants and creatures, the Garden of Eden was also created, and it was into this earthly paradise that Adam and Eve were brought forth. It is recorded that they were both naked and thus they were no different from the other animals. The first humans would not want for food, since the garden supplied them with every plant or tree bearing seed or fruit, the fish in the sea, the fowl of the air, and "every living thing that moveth upon the earth". You would think that the couple would have been content with their lot, adopting a carefree lifestyle of foraging in a landscape of plenty. However, they chose to disobey the one contrary instruction they had been given – that is, do not eat the fruit of the Tree of Knowledge. As a direct result of this act of disobedience, they were expelled from the Garden of Eden. No longer could they rely on the garden to provide them with their food, so henceforth their children, Cain and Abel, would have to work much harder for their living, either by tilling the ground to grow crops or by herding livestock. This, then, is the curious tale of the expulsion from Eden. It is an ancient myth recording a divine punishment visited upon the first foraging humans, forcing their offspring to learn the complex and unpredictable principles of crop farming and animal husbandry.

Scientists in the 21st century now have a clearer and far more precise view of how life on earth evolved, when the human race first appeared on the scene and the long development of its characteristic foraging culture. These are the lengthy eras later termed the Old and Middle Stone Age, or the Palaeolithic or Mesolithic periods: we can identify them metaphorically with the Garden of Eden. But for how long have we been, genetically speaking, foraging in the garden? How old is the human race, and for how long have we had the mindset of hunter-gatherers (like the proverbial Adam and Eve) programmed into our genes?

Trying to trace our ancestors is an almost universal interest – most of us want to know where we've come from. But as we try to compile the family tree, many of us discover that it's hard to find clear evidence of a connection beyond our great-great grandparents. This is because we usually have to rely on the written evidence provided by, for example, registers of births, marriages and deaths or surviving census returns. Unfortunately, the full range of such documents rarely survives for the 17th or 18th century, and so our search all too often comes to an abrupt end. For many of us, our historical and emotional memory is only about 200 or 300 years. It is increasingly hard to empathise strongly with our more distant ancestors, those for whom we have no photographs and rarely even any names. Luckily, recent advances in scientific research have provided new routes to follow, and these can take us back thousands, indeed millions, of years into our past. Archaeology can show us how we lived in our deep past, while the study of genetics and DNA can tell us very precisely who our direct but distant relations actually were. Using research from both these avenues, the broad lines of our most distant history can be plotted, an approach that identifies aspects of our lives today which we have unwittingly inherited from our Palaeolithic past.

The Venerable Bede, a monk researching the Holy Bible in a Northumbrian monastery in the eighth century AD, suggested that the world was created just under 6,000 years ago, in about 3952 BC. The Christian monks in late ninth-century Winchester traced the ancestry of the Saxon King Æthelwulf back to Hratha (a direct descendant of Adam) who was born on Noah's ark (Garmonsway 1972, 66). Thus, they estimated that the world was created rather earlier, in about 5195 BC (Garmonsway 1972, 28). Working through the genealogies listed in the Old Testament in the late 17th century, Archbishop Usher provided some precision to this long-running debate, famously declaring that the creation of the world could be dated to Sunday 23 October 4004 BC.

Alas, the work of those scholars was rudely overturned by the research of geologists such as James Hutton (1785) and Charles Lyell (1833). Their study of rock formations subsequently showed that the earth was, in fact, very much older than that, as were the origins of animal and plant life on the planet. However, the date when the first humans appeared was still open to question. Scholars were finding and starting to study ancient artefacts, and in Europe at least, C. J. Thomsen had classified them into three period-based groups, the youngest being termed the Iron Age, which was later than the Bronze Age, with the oldest artefacts termed Stone Age (Thomsen 1848). The ancient material could now be seen in a relative sequence to which later scholars would then apply increasingly more accurate dating.

The next big breakthrough came in the momentous year of 1859, with studies by Joseph Prestwich and John Evans in England and by Boucher de Perthes in France. Their archaeological excavations revealed stone hand axes made by humans lying in the same layers as the bones of long extinct animals, known to have died out many thousands of years *before* 4004 BC. Clearly, humans were at least as old as sabre-toothed tigers, but precisely how much older were they?

Directed or undirected evolution?

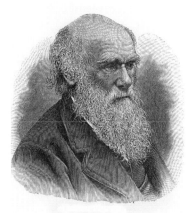

Charles Darwin (1809–1882).

We have summarised how the human race evolved from its humble primate origins to take the form of anatomically modern humans (that is, us) and mastery over the whole planet. It's worth stressing that the form we take now was not preordained or predetermined: it is no more than the chance conjunction of attributes and mutations which the survivors in an ever-changing world passed on to us. It is illogical to assume that the blind but powerful forces of nature that provided ice ages, continental drift and supported dinosaurs for 135 million years (far, far longer than us) had a master plan specifically for the development of *Homo sapiens*. Left to its own unreasoning devices, nature's evolutionary paths are essentially undirected (Stringer and Andrews 2011, 226), although they do progress within a set of (often conflicting) parameters, the outcomes of which can be suggested (rather than predicted) with varying degrees of certainty.

Natural selection is therefore undirected, since it is not consciously working towards a specific goal or physiological form. If a particular genetic configuration cannot adapt to a changing environment, then the lineage will die out: ostensibly a simple case of survival or extinction. The long process which culminated in the appearance of *Homo sapiens* less than 200,000 years ago was not part of a preconceived master plan. We mutated from tree-living, fruit-eating quadrupeds into ground-living bipedal omnivores not because the earth necessarily needed such creatures, nor even that there was an empty niche in the natural pecking order that *Homo sapiens* felt obliged to fill. It was just the unplanned product of a curious conjunction of evolutionary and climatic circumstance. New fold mountains were not formed because there was a progressive evolutionary need for them, but because continents collided. Our bodies and our minds were similarly uplifted through the arbitrary conjunction of colliding circumstances.

Fate, happenstance and good (or ill) fortune all played a part in our evolutionary journey. For a start, our ancestors were (unlike plants or mountain ranges) sentient creatures, hence the term *Homo sapiens*. They could and did have an unwitting hand in their own unpredictable future through the basic process of sexual selection: how a male or female chooses a particular partner to mate with. The choice, if choice there was, might rest on simple availability (a real problem with small isolated tribal groupings) as much as on perceived characteristics. At one end of a very wide spectrum is mutual attraction; at the far end lies alpha male dominance, perhaps with many partners, willing or otherwise, related or otherwise. The offspring of such unions, complete with the genetic inheritance of both partners, therefore provides a biased gene pool, the raw material upon which the more mechanistic laws of natural selection would only then be brought to bear.

Thus the somewhat arbitrary course of sexual selection produced the somewhat arbitrary gene pool from which only the fittest would survive. The breeding generation this produced was then subjected to another round of arbitrary sexual selection. It is perfectly possible that many millennia ago different unions of males and females could have produced a radically different human gene pool: stronger or weaker, more or less gifted, more or less adaptable than we became. It could have turned out so differently, as the ignominious fate of the now extinct *Homo neanderthalensis* or *Homo floresiensis* graphically shows. Rather than through purposeful evolution, it was by a combination of chance mutations, adaptions and gene flow between Neanderthals and anatomically modern humans, as well as pure happenstance, that *Homo sapiens* eventually became the successful hunter-gathering colonist of five continents.

So much for undirected evolution. Directed evolution, by contrast, is also possible – as anyone involved with the breeding of racehorses or roses can confirm – by conscious and considered selection of the specimens allowed to procreate. Darwin himself was much involved in the breeding and cross-breeding of pigeons to develop particular traits. This, he fully appreciated, was an artificial, fast-track intervention in a complex genetic process – "variation under domestication": humans were simply manipulating blind biological processes for their own ends to 'improve' on nature. Directed evolution produced a better pigeon; undirected evolution produced the urbanised human.

Our lowly origins

Charles Darwin's pioneering study of evolution laid the foundations for the next phase of research, with his major works *On the Origin of Species* (1859) and *The Descent of Man* (1871). In the 'Historical Sketch' that prefaces his introduction to *On the Origin of Species*, Darwin discusses opinions commonly held before the publication of his own landmark volume. It includes comments by his grandfather, Dr Erasmus Darwin, noted in *Zoonomia* (1794), as well as some by the celebrated naturalist Lamarck (1830) through to the paper presented at the Linnaean Society on 1 July 1858 by Alfred Russel Wallace, Professor Thomas Henry Huxley's lecture to the Royal Institution in June 1859 and Dr Joseph Dalton Hooker's Introduction to the Australian Flora of the same year (Hooker 1859). The evidence presented demonstrated that all the wide varieties of flora and fauna on the planet with which we are familiar today (including humans) were not all created ready-made on the same day. Not only that, but it was now proving possible to trace the progenitors of many species back to their ancestral forms.

It was then suggested that the human race (*Homo sapiens*) and the African great apes share a common primate ancestor, and thus a common place of birth. In this Darwin was building on the work of, for example, the English physician Edward Tyson, whose publication on the dissection of a chimpanzee in 1699 noted that the anatomy was similar to our own. Subsequently, Thomas Henry Huxley asserted that humans should be placed in the same order as apes (Huxley 1863). This was the same year that the study of fossil hominid species began, with William King's presentation of the proposed *Homo neanderthalensis* to the British Association (see Johanson and Edgar 1996, 228). Thus, the lowly origins of humanity were gradually revealed, to the consternation and disbelief of an unsuspecting world.

How and why these organisms changed, mutated and developed into their current guise is a second crucial question. According to Darwin, 'natural selection' was a key process that adjudicated in the continuing immutable struggle with nature against famine and death. It served as the agency that selects the fittest progeny that would survive and procreate (and therefore which inherited attributes would be passed on) and which would be rendered extinct.

In biological terms, Darwinian evolution is a long-term process of genetic change, often in mechanistic response to the pressures of external factors including environmental change, natural predators, disease, accidents and the varying potential and size of the available gene pool. His concept of natural selection (i.e. the survival of the fittest) is based on at least three issues. First there is *genetic heredity*: individuals can only inherit the basket of genetic traits that their parents had (e.g. eye or hair colour, shape of ears and nose and other physiological features) and that assemblage will exclude all traits not incorporated in their respective genomes. The second issue is that there is a considerable number of such *gene variants* in any population, suggesting many possible future permutations for future progeny. Then there is the problem of *differential reproduction*: not all individuals will get to reproduce successfully, while some will reproduce more than others, sometimes with different partners. But what of the fate of the children of the children of such unions, with their own mixture of hereditary genetic traits (or genotype)?

According to Darwin, this is where the processes of natural selection begin to operate: the survival of the fittest. Biologists use the term 'fitness' to describe how a particular genotype would ultimately survive and reproduce successfully, in comparison with its contemporaries. Obviously, fitness is a relative term since so much depends on the contemporary environment: the fittest genotype during an ice age, for example, may not have been the fittest genotype once the glaciers had retreated. The fittest individual was thus not necessarily the strongest, the best looking, the biggest or the most intelligent: it simply refers to the ability to survive at a particular time and place, find a consensual (or non-consensual) mate and produce offspring that would themselves survive and reproduce. The lineages that subsequently died out took with them their own individual genetic traits; consequently the wider population enjoyed less genetic variation than before. Nevertheless, even Darwin appreciated that, although natural selection was of prime importance, it was "not the exclusive means of modification" (Darwin 1859, 23): sexual selection, genetic mutation and even pure chance also had roles to play in our evolutionary story, as will be shown.

Blood brothers and sisters

Distant cousins

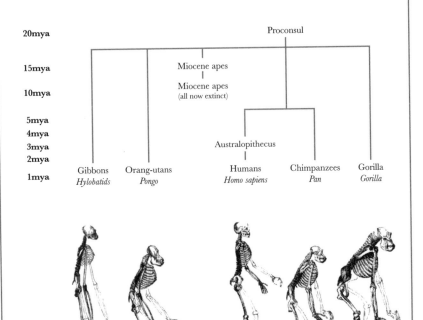

20mya   Proconsul

15mya   Miocene apes

10mya   Miocene apes
(all now extinct)

5mya
4mya
3mya   Australopithecus
2mya

1mya   Gibbons   Orang-utans   Humans   Chimpanzees   Gorilla
      Hylobatids   *Pongo*   *Homo sapiens*   *Pan*   *Gorilla*

GIBBON.   ORANG.   MAN.   CHIMPANZEE.   GORILLA.

*Photographically reduced from Diagrams of the natural size (except that of the Gibbon, which was twice as large as nature),
drawn by Mr. Waterhouse Hawkins from specimens in the Museum of the Royal College of Surgeons.*

Our near relations: frontispiece in Thomas Henry Huxley's
Evidence as to Man's Place in Nature (1863).

This summary diagram shows our present understanding of the last 20 million years of our long evolution from the time of our great-great ancestor, the family of apes called Proconsul, to the present day.

Proconsuls were also the distant but directly related ancestors of today's gorillas, orang-utans, gibbons and chimpanzees. These creatures are therefore our genetic relations; indeed, our closest relatives in this table are chimpanzees, with whom we share 98% of our genetic make-up.

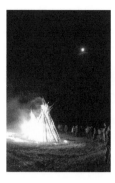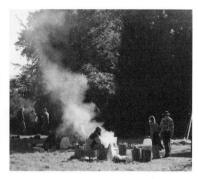

Figure 2.2. Nothing like an open fire: domestication of fire transformed the hunter-gatherers' world, providing warmth, security (left) and facility to cook otherwise indigestible foodstuffs (right).

Ascent of man

Armed with the principles of undirected evolutionary development and a grounding in archaeological research and genetic studies, an attempt can be made to sketch in key moments of change in our deep and distant past. In 1984, a study by Charles Sibley and Jon Ahlquist initially suggested that chimpanzee and human genomes are 98.4% similar: clearly they shared a common ancestor at some period in their past. Work has also progressed on the nature of the differences between them, with, for example, Svante Pääbo reporting that a gene important in speech articulation (FOXP2) differed significantly (Enard et al. 2002). Meanwhile, the National Human Genome Research Institute in the United States continued its ground-breaking studies of DNA sequences from humans and chimpanzees, and published its initial findings between 2003 and 2005 (Nature 2005).

Research since then has seen the publication of the genome of the macaque in 2007 and of the orang-utan in 2011, with studies of the bonobo, gorilla and baboon all underway. We are therefore unravelling not just our own evolutionary history with greater scientific clarity, but we can also illuminate our distant (and not so distant) relationship with the other primates. The recent publication by the geneticist Eugene Harris from New York University's Center for the Study of Human Origins summarises much of the work in this pioneering field, providing the hard evidence for Darwin's visionary views (Harris 2014).

Dysfunctional family?

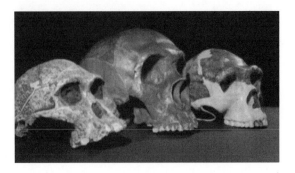

Changing faces: restored fossil skulls of ancestral humans.

Seven million years of evolution, adaption and mutation: the disjointed, diverse and diverging family tree of the ape lineage that includes us, the anatomically modern humans. All the discrete fossil finds listed here are linked genetically in some way, but the precise parentage and verified links between them is still the focus of fierce debate. More well-dated specimens must be discovered before our most ancient genealogy can be more firmly established, but this table shows the approximate age and chronology of some of our more famous ancestors. It seems that progeny of the Australopithecine line ultimately produced at least 11 branches of the 'human' family. Most of these subsequently died out, leaving just *Homo sapiens* that still survives today.

7mya			
		Sahelanthropus tchadensis	
6mya			
		Orrorin tugenesis	
		Ardipithecus kadabba	
5mya			
		Ardipithecus ramidus	
		Australopithecus anamensis	
4mya			
	Kenyanthropus platypos		*Australopithecus afarensis*
3mya			
		Paranthropus aethiopicus	
	Australopithecus africanus		*Australopithecus gahri*
2mya		**HUMANS**	
	Homo rudolfensis		*Homo habilis*
	Homo erectus	*Australopithecus sediba*	*Paranthropus robustus*
1mya		*Homo naledi*	
	Homo antecessor		*Homo ergaster*
	Homo neanderthalensis		*Homo heidelbergensis*
	Denisovans		*Homo floresiensis*

Six to eight million years ago: a common ancestor

According to this crucial DNA evidence and further archaeological studies, a much clearer picture is slowly beginning to emerge. We now know not only how old we humans are, but also that our gene stock can be traced back well beyond our ancient past to an ancestral line shared with other primates well over seven million years ago (Andrews 2015). It seems that all these primates were foragers, a trait in our genetic make-up that is actually substantially older – that is to say, millions of years older – than humanity itself. These creatures, our ancestors, do not seem to have enjoyed the powers of reasoning and intellect of modern humans, but relied on instincts and basic emotional drives instead. Many of the earliest primates spent much of their lives in the trees, where climbing and swinging from branches was the standard mode of propulsion, using their well-developed arms to move them from branch to branch. When on the ground, our ancestors would normally walk or run on all fours, quite unlike how we move today. When did all this change?

Three to five million years ago: human-like

The last common ancestor of humans and chimpanzees still moved on four legs, but we can now suggest that the two lineages that became either apes or humans began to separate out about six million years ago, since the oldest fossil remains that resemble bipedal humans date to this period. Research at Harvard University in Boston has provided some evidence of interbreeding over the next four million years, however, as the female (X) chromosomes were still so similar (Patterson et al. 2006). But fossilised footprints found at Laetoli in Tanzania prove conclusively that human ancestors were walking upright, using just their hind legs, some four million years ago. The new creatures which had identifiable 'human' characteristics were not simple fruit or plant eaters (fructivores or herbivores) but ate a more mixed diet (omnivores) that incorporated meat in various forms (e.g. animals, fish, birds, insects). They include *Ardipithecus ramidus*, appearing some 4.5 million years ago and *Australopithecus afarensis* some three million years ago. Recent fieldwork has recovered stone tools from the shores of Lake Turkana in Kenya. These date back some 3.3 million years, and are thus the oldest such items found anywhere in the world. Even more dramatically, they are older than the oldest fossil representative of the genus *Homo* yet recorded. So is stone tool technology (often regarded as representing the first material evidence of the long march to civilisation) actually earlier than the evolution of the creatures we now call humans?

500,000 to 2.6 million years ago: becoming human

The somewhat later stone tools recovered in Olduvai Gorge in Tanzania from deposits dated to 2.6 million years ago could have been used either by the later generations of the Australopithecines or *Homo habilis*, the earliest members of our very own genus. Some of the branches in the ancient human family tree may have coexisted, rather than replaced each other directly, such as *Homo habilis* who may have lived between 2.6 and 1.5 million years ago. It was in this period that there seems to have been a change in skull shape and size. This saw a significant increase in the capacity of the cranium which suggests an increased brain size (Mithen 1996, 11–12).

Acheulean hand axes are complex worked stone implements, and the oldest examples discovered so far are the 1.76-million-year-old examples from Lake Turkana (Kenya) found in 2011. The technology and culture represented by these finds arguably lasted for over one million years, and was so long lived and so widespread as to demonstrate that those early humans not only learned the skills to make them but were also able to share that ability with many others – all very human traits. These hand axes are broadly contemporary with more significant anatomical developments, which sees the gradual selection of the characteristic features now seen as representing *Homo erectus* or *Homo ergaster*, from about 1.8 million years ago. This species had a smaller gut and smaller molar teeth but a larger brain than *Homo habilis*, perhaps implying a keener mind, improved communication skills and greater ability to respond to change.

All of the data on our early development come from Africa (Rightmire 2009), with the first evidence of the hominid colonisation of Europe only occurring some 1.3 million years ago in southern Spain. This was a time when sea levels in the Straits of Gibraltar were up to 100 metres lower than today, allowing a range of animals to migrate northwards. As for the prehistory of Great Britain, the earliest evidence of human remains have been recovered from sites such as Boxgrove in Sussex (Stringer 2006). Here the partial tibia of a male *Homo heidelbergensis* who probably stood 1.8 metres high and weighed around 80 kg were found on the site in 1994, while two incisor teeth from another individual were found two years later on a site that produced many flint tools and animal bones dating to 500,000 before present (BP) (Roberts and Parfitt 1999).

10,000 to 500,000 years ago: human beings

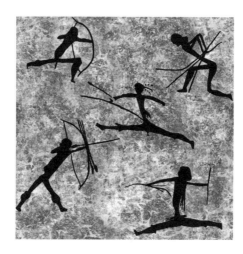

Figure 2.3. Cave painting: images of
Palaeolithic hunters from Lascaux, France.

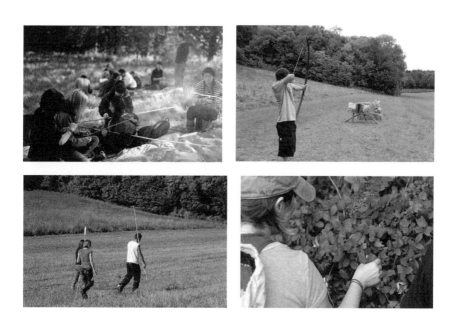

Figure 2.4. Object lessons in hunter-gathering – UCL
Institute of Archaeology Field School: (a) making spears,
(b) target practice with a bow and arrow, (c) a hunting
party sets off and (d) gathering hedgerow fruits.

The oldest remains yet recorded of the anatomically modern human *Homo sapiens* have been found in Israel, dating back some 400,000 BP, according to a report by Professor Avi Gopher and Dr Ran Barkai of the Institute of Archaeology at Tel Aviv University (Stiner et al. 2010). This is substantially older than the otherwise similar material discovered in Middle Awash, Ethiopia, in deposits from *c.*160,000 BP.

Homo sapiens may have coexisted, at least for a while, with the much misunderstood Neanderthals (*Homo neanderthalensis*), who had large crania and were accomplished stone tool makers. However, genetic material from a 45,000-year-old male Neanderthal specimen found in Vindija Cave outside Zagreb, was analysed by geneticist Svante Pääbo's team (Pääbo 2014). This work showed marked differences from that of modern humans and also from chimpanzee Y chromosomes. Even more significant is the re-evaluation of the dating of sites and sequences across Europe: John Hawks (University of Wisconsin–Madison) and William Davies (Centre for the Archaeology of Human Origins, University of Southampton) both argue against any significant settlement overlap between Neanderthals and modern humans. It now seems *Homo sapiens* adapted faster and more effectively to the changing climatic conditions than their older rivals: there were no prizes for coming second.

In addition to the Neanderthals, more of the ultimately less successful branches of the family tree have been discovered. Artefacts and animal bones have been recovered from a long sequence of occupation deposits in a cave in the Altai Mountains in Siberia, along with some human remains, some of which can be dated from 30,000 to 48,000 BP. A female finger bone from this site has been examined at the Max Planck Institute for Evolutionary Anthropology at Leipzig by a team led by Johannes Krause. According to a report in the journal *Nature*, the study of the mitochondrial DNA suggests that the 'X-woman' represented may be a new species, *Denisova hominin*, rather than a Neanderthal (Reich et al. 2010). For reasons that will be long debated, both these lines became extinct – the same fate shared by the diminutive creature known as *Homo floresiensis*, the remains of which were recently discovered in Indonesia where they were living in splendid isolation until some 12,000 years ago.

Perhaps one of the most unusual excavations of a prehistoric site took place in 2013 in the Dinaledi Chamber, a claustrophobic cave in South Africa, directed by Lee Berger of the University of Witwatersrand (Berger et al. 2015). The site was so constrictive that a team of six 'skinny and small' excavators had to be specially recruited to penetrate to the bottom of the shaft before recording and recovering an assemblage of 1,550 bone fragments from at least 15 individuals. It is argued that a possible new hominin species is represented, initially described as *Homo naledi*, but the dating at perhaps about 100,000 BP is at present unconfirmed and unclear.

The period in which *Homo sapiens* subsequently colonised the continents has been marked by a continuation in a dramatically oscillating climatic pattern, with major glacial advances and subsequent retreats (interglacials): it was not just that the temperatures changed but, of course, so too did the flora and fauna, the very world of the hunter-gatherer. Adaptability was, as ever, the key to survival: the only other path led to extinction. Indeed, of all the human variants summarily discussed here, only *Homo sapiens* currently survives.

Archaeologists have thus studied the skeletal remains, settlements sites, arte-facts and food remains of our direct ancestors in various parts of the world. From this accumulating database, it is possible to establish where and how they lived and the variations on the hunter-gatherer regimes they used to survive over this long period. Research has also turned to more abstract issues, such as how they interacted socially and how language may have developed. This all relates to the evolution of more stimulating thought processes.

In this continuing study of our deep cultural evolution, the development of traits like cave painting, more specialised hunting techniques and the pro-duction of objects such as Venus figurines are seen as highly significant and interrelated. They seem to form part of what has been termed a 'creative explosion'. Research over the last 20 years on material from South Africa, North Africa and the Levant suggests that the earliest traces of this profound advance may be found in Africa, perhaps as long ago as 250,000 BP. There is now considerable evidence for such developments between 70,000 and 100,000 BP in other regions, and especially around 45,000 BP. Increased communication and understanding through rhythmic, verbal and visual media – that is, through music in various forms, through rudimentary speech and through art – all had their roles to play in bonding, informing and developing these Palaeolithic societies.

All such developments would have a part to play in the successful survival of communities, in sexual selection and thus in directed and undirected evolu-tion of our physiology and culture. We can therefore plot the development not just of our biological evolution, but also of cultural changes over that vast period, as well as the significant interactions of those two trajectories. Taken together, these three strands of biology, culture and, crucially, their interactive co-adaption, form the complex interwoven story of what has been called human evolution.

5,000 to 10,000 years ago: from foraging to farming

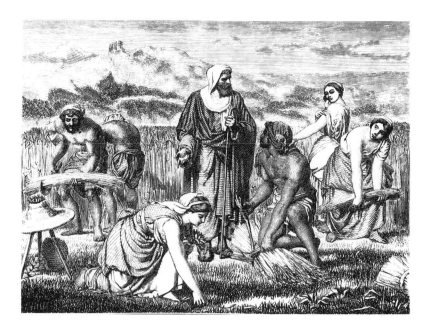

Figure 2.5. Agriculture in antiquity: growing managed cereals involved clearing fields, ploughing, sowing seeds and then harvesting the crop – a very labour-intensive operation.

As these early human communities gradually spread outwards from their ancestral lands in Africa to the other continents, they adapted differing forms of hunter-gatherer cultures to better fit the new environments they encountered. For thousands of years, such cultures developed and adapted to a changing climate, changing terrain and changing flora and fauna.

The next questions to be answered are these: when, and why, did we stop living as hunter-gatherers? Arguably these were the most significant changes in human cultural evolution and had a profound effect on our later development. Given that necessity is frequently the mother of invention, the key drivers of climate change and population pressure must have had a role to play, but it is clear that the transition developed in different regions at different dates; indeed, a few isolated areas have still not wholly adopted modernity today.

It was not until some 5,000 to 10,000 years ago that the first forms of recognisable 'farming' developed. This is reflected in the dating for the earliest evidence for the domestication of particular plants and livestock, the period referred to as the Neolithic or New Stone Age. This saw the conscious, directed evolution of crops through selective planting and animals through selective breeding. Greater control over food resources led, in theory if not always in practice, to the support of more densely populated communities and regions, and thus larger and potentially more varied gene pools. The impact of natural selection on humanity was thereby lessened.

The most recent research suggests that there were perhaps as many as six foci where these new, more intensive agricultural regimes were tried, tested and developed independently. From these centres, the ideas spread by imitation, migration or invasion. The earliest evidence comes from the Fertile Crescent (in modern-day Iraq) from 11,000 BP. It may be significant that this is the region through which the Tigris and Euphrates rivers flow, both of which are also mentioned by name in the biblical account of the Garden of Eden (Genesis 2:10–14), as an article on the research of Dr Juris Zarins published in the *Smithsonian Magazine* (see Hamblin 1997) suggests. However, there were other such 'Edens' in which the new farming practices supplanted the older hunter-gathering regimes. One was the region in China that included the Yangtze and Yellow River basins, where the Neolithic Revolution had begun by at least 9,000 BP; another was in the New Guinea Highlands between 9,000–6,000 BP. The earliest such developments from eastern sub-Saharan Africa may date rather later to 5,000–4,000 BP, and a similar date range is recorded for Central Mexico and northern South America, with evidence from the United States dating to 4,000–3,000 BP.

The story in Europe can be related to its complex genetic population history, which is an obvious mixture of many ancestral strands. The recovery and analysis of DNA from the bones of prehistoric skeletons has already thrown light on three key strands in the story of the hunter-gatherer colonisation of the continent. In 2015, a team from Trinity College Dublin identified a fourth group that has contributed to our European DNA. They were initially isolated in the Caucasus but later seem to have migrated eastwards. Taken together, it now seems that the first hunter-gatherers, Group A, migrated out of Africa, probably travelled through Turkey and into Europe around 45,000 years ago. Group B settled in the Caucasus, but were isolated from all other groups around 25,000 years ago, according to the new research. A third group, who had settled in the Levant, seem to have participated in the development of the new Neolithic agricultural methods, and then moved across Europe with these game-changing practices some 6,000 to 7,000 years ago. By then, Group B had interbred with other human groups from further east, which ultimately became incorporated into the Yamnaya culture, Group D, who then migrated into Europe, probably from the Altai Mountains around 5,000 years ago, and possibly introduced the Proto-Indo-European language (Jones et al. 2015).

The crops that initially became the focus of the new Neolithic practices were cereals such as strains of wheat (e.g. emmer and einkorn) and barley, which fared well in the Mediterranean climate with its short rainy seasons and long hot summers to ripen the large seeds. Such cereals required considerable processing before producing something that the human gut could actually digest, but in spite of the extra effort involved, bread became a staple food, even though it is less nutritious than the raw materials on the forager's table. There is evidence from the Jordan Valley for the cultivation of barley, oats and figs, in parts of Asia rice became the staple, while bananas and plantains may have been first cultivated in New Guinea. In Africa, a range of crops from differing eco-zones were husbanded, including coffee, millet, sorghum, yams, kola nuts and the oil palm. On the other side of the Pacific, corn, beans, squash and then maize were grown in Mesoamerica, potatoes and manioc in South America, and sunflower, sumpweed and goosefoot in the eastern United States. Women may have had a special role to play in the new programmes of cultivation, rather than solely collecting wild products when ripe. Their localised but deep botanical observation and knowledge – essential to all gatherers – would have certainly been a key stepping stone in the process.

Loss of innocence

Whatever the trigger, the rigours of the long daily expedition to comb the countryside for edible products in season could be supplemented, and then largely replaced, by harvesting the presumably more predictable gardens, allotments or fields that were closer at hand. The labour involved for those first 'farmers' (or perhaps market gardeners?) was considerable, but the effort invested produced a higher return. The settlements or small holdings that grew up around these fields developed more as permanent villages, rather than as temporary, mobile camp-sites.

As a consequence of this more settled, sedentary approach, the role of the hunter also began changing. Rather than hunting parties tracking herbivores over vast distances or intercepting them at key points on an annual migration, the concept gradually developed of 'domesticating' animals into herds that could be culled as required. Sheep, goats, cows and pigs were among the earliest animals domesticated for food, as well as for the by-products such as leather and wool. How such initially wild animals were duly tamed is also debated: orphans whose parents had been killed in the hunt may have been one source, while the universal ability of children (or at least those who are not hungry) to adopt injured creatures is another.

Animals also had other uses, so dogs, camels, llamas, oxen and horses were also put to work, as were the ancestors of domestic fowl and other birds. There was, however, a downside to living too closely with animals, and that was the risk of diseases such as influenza, smallpox and measles spreading to humans. Just as sedentary settlements and society started to grow, so too did infectious and contagious diseases, often with devastating consequences. Only those with a natural immunity to these attacks, perhaps only a small minority, would be strong enough to survive and procreate.

In many parts of the world, fundamental changes in the daily lives of the former hunter-gathering societies could thus be seen, although the changes were uncoordinated and spread out over several thousand years and many generations. Not all succeeded, for there could be reverses if there were major crop failures, demanding a return to an older regime. (Inuit hunters took over the lands of the failed Scandinavian farmers in areas like Greenland, for example.) Nevertheless, over large areas of the globe in the space of a few thousand years, there was a Neolithic Revolution: the 'new' systems of animal husbandry and crop cultivation it introduced gradually changed not just our diet but also the sorts of settlement and society in which we could live. We could support a much larger, more diverse population now that we had developed greater control over our food supply, but we seemed to have far less control over our health or security.

Life before farming depended on the bounty of nature and living symbiotically with it. By contrast, life for the new farmers, and the societies they supported, depended increasingly on their own ingenuity – these new communities were, more than ever, responsible for their own fate. Archaeologists today are in agreement that this fundamental change, this transition from foraging to farming, was probably the single most crucial development in human cultural progress. It brought in its wake the need for territories with fixed boundaries in the landscape to protect fields, resources and settlements, while the ever larger concentrated populations that could now be fed saw the rise of towns, states and empires.

These later phases of development, with the associated rise in population numbers, invariably impacted upon the social structure. Small tribal societies, by their nature, are ones in which the names of all are known by all. In a larger urban settlement, the names and personalities of the many all too often disappear. A large society also requires an elite, a hierarchy and often a rigid organisation if it is to run smoothly. Thus, following on from the domestication of plants and animals, the larger towns and empires required greater social stratification, including an underclass. Thus the Neolithic Revolution also led to the domestication of humans (or at least those that were deemed the lesser sort), with the evolution of a landless, labouring or slave class, without which such monuments as the Egyptian pyramids could not have been built.

Chapter 3

A VIEW OF THE GARDEN

… as free as Nature first made man …

When wild in woods the noble Savage ran.

John Dryden (1631–1700)

Hunter-gatherers

What exactly is a Noble Savage? From the comfort of our centrally heated urban homes we can speculate on just how uncivilised we used to be, in the dark and distant days before civilisation dawned. How noble were we then, and how savage were our lifestyles? We tend to categorise the cultures adopted by ancient Palaeolithic populations using such catch-all terms as hunter-gatherer (as opposed to farmer or city dweller), but it is as well to appreciate that they would not have described themselves in those terms. For them, living off the land was a given: daily life centred round the acquisition of sufficient food and water to see them through the day. The next meal could be trapped, snared, shot, fished, picked, plucked, dug up or chopped down: it all depended on the season and the terrain.

All this shows how adaptable and resourceful the human race needed to be. Regardless of climatic zone or contours, it seems that our pioneering ancestors could carve a survival niche in almost any landscape, from the most welcoming to the dramatically harsh, should circumstances demand it. Indeed, up until c.AD 1500, about one-third of the global land mass was still occupied by un-urbanised hunter-gatherers, some far from 'civilisation', while others were living on the very edge of encroaching modernity (Lee and Daly 1999, 405). Even the youthful English gentleman Charles Darwin was able to observe "naked savages in their native lands" in Tierra del Fuego during his voyages to the far corners of the known world on HMS *Beagle* between 1831 and 1836.

It is difficult to sum up several millennia of regionally diverse cultures in a few sentences, but some of the key common elements should be stressed. Some communities lived in the tropics, while others survived the rigours of an ice age. Each region had its own ecosystem, its own range of seasonally changing plant and animal life. They also proffered very real dangers, since each continent bred wild and wily carnivores. Long-term survival in such extremely diverse environments required detailed knowledge of what plants, nuts, berries and roots could or could not be eaten (and, crucially, when they could or could not be eaten), which creatures could or could not be eaten, and which ones might want to eat you. Such knowledge could not be acquired instantly, but major mistakes would be fatal. Our ancestors had to be fast learners and good teachers. They also had to be mobile, since for many, home was where the food was: the camp-sites moved with the seasons to keep pace with migrating herds or to adapt to changes in climate, vegetation or sea levels. They were thus very physically active: running or walking long distances daily was the norm, as was the carrying of heavy loads, the making of tools, the preparation of meals and the building of houses and shelters.

To be effective exponents of such wilderness living requires successful social interaction. Knowledge of the territory and its resources needed to be learned and shared, hunting parties depended heavily on each other, foraging groups worked as teams of young and not so young. All members of the community contributed towards the common good, with little room for passengers. Young men might make the best hunters; older women might be the most experienced botanists. Identification with your tribe, your territory, was not a matter of patriotic choice; it was a question of survival.

An ethnographic perspective

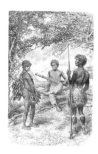 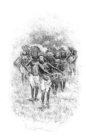 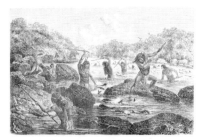

Figure 3.1. Team work: hunter-gatherer cultures involve the whole community if sufficient food is to be found each day, as these three images of plant collection and spear fishing show.

Having established that the human race survived for a long time as hunter-gatherers – in our proverbial Eden – it would be instructive to know just what such a regime was like on a daily basis. Superficially, it seems to bear little or no relationship to modern city life, although subsequent chapters will show how not much has changed at a deeper level. The details of how such ancient foraging communities lived and worked can be reconstructed in outline, as Chapters 3 and 4 will show.

This can then be supplemented and greatly extended by recent ethnographic and anthropological studies of communities in those few corners of the world neglected or untouched by large-scale agriculture and urbanisation (e.g. Schrire 1984; Cummings et al. 2014). These indigenous peoples developed – and are still developing – their own individual survival regimes in very different settings. There is no reason to assume that the techniques and cultural practices exhibited today need be identical to those the region may have seen in previous millennia, although it seems clear that some of the basic concepts and approaches could boast a considerable antiquity. The following examples are presented to provide no more than a broad-brush illustration of some of the great variety of ways in which ancient hunter-gatherer communities may have operated.

Tiwi

Our journey will start in the southern hemisphere, with the reports about the Tiwi made by C. M. W. Hart in 1928–1929 (Hart et al. 1988, 147–162). The islands of Bathurst and Melville lie off the northern coast of Australia, some 50 to 80 miles from Darwin. By the 18th and early 19th century, these islands were populated by the Tiwi tribe, all of whom lived as hunter-gatherers, a regime that archaeologists have traced back some 30,000 years in this area. There were nine named bands, each of between 100 and 300 people, who roamed around a 'territory' of some 200 to 300 square miles from which they fed themselves. The territory was their 'country' and the band was their 'own people'. Nevertheless, all nine bands spoke the same language, and kinship and other alliances were possible and prevalent between them.

Each band was subdivided into 'households', extended family groups which made their own decisions as to where and when they would set up camp and forage within their own territory. Their mobility related directly to food sources and seasonality, and thus 'permanent' homes did not exist, just a succession of temporary camp-sites. Every day the men would set out at daybreak for the hunt. Such an exercise is never totally predictable, and requires teamwork, speed, agility, patience and a thorough knowledge of the creatures and their particular habitats if it is to be successful. For the Tiwi, the prey ranged from large lizards, kangaroos and other marsupials from the inland areas, to wild geese, fish, turtles and dugongs from the coast or rivers. These foods were highly prized, but were nevertheless a bonus, for the staple products were those collected, carried and processed by the women: nuts, fruits, vegetables and tubers. The kwoka nuts from the local palm trees, for example, were collected in quantity when in season, then soaked and pounded into a porridge-like dish. During January and February it was the turn of a yam called the kulama to provide the staple, its abundance providing the basis for collective tribal ceremonial feasts timed to coincide with this particular harvest. It was thus on the detailed knowledge of the older women, who knew the vegetation and productive cycle of their lands so intimately, that the long-term prosperity of the household depended. The younger women had much to learn before they would be as highly prized.

A varied and nutritious diet was thus shaped by the seasons, the landscape itself, the chance finds of the hunter and the more predictable staples gathered by the women. Without refrigerators, there was a requirement to forage every day of the week, unless food could be stored, dried or otherwise preserved. That said, the Tiwi on these well-watered islands lived well above starvation levels through practising a hunter-gathering regime that they and their ancestors gradually developed over a 30,000-year period (Hart et al. 1988).

Inuit

One of the key components in the story of human evolution is adaptability; as Darwin pointed out, it is not necessarily the strongest or most intelligent that survive, but the most adaptable. Consequently, not all hunter-gatherer regimes are by any means the same, since survival in contrasting continents requires a detailed knowledge of each particular landscape. The subarctic region peopled by the Inuit is a world away from the subtropical Australian coast, but still supported a regime similar in principle to that of the Tiwi but vastly different in practice. Perhaps the biggest difference is that there was little in the way of plant matter to collect in their environment; therefore, for most of the year they were hunter-fishers rather than hunter-gatherers.

The tree-less region stretching from Alaska, USA, and Newfoundland, Canada, to Greenland has been occupied by the Inuit, Inupiat and Yupik since at least the Middle Ages. In an area where crops simply could not be grown, the Inuit had no option but to survive through hunting and fishing. Whales, seals, walruses and seabirds were regular prey, as were caribou, musk-oxen and even polar bears. Again, seasonal migrations to particular locations and habitats would be required and, when available, the diet would be augmented by vegetable matter, such as grasses, tubers, roots and seaweed.

For the Inuit, 75% of their daily energy intake came from fat, a very different situation from the Tiwi. In the 1920s, the anthropologist Vilhjalmur Stefansson (1946) studied the Inuit's extremely low-carbohydrate diet, and reported that it had no adverse effects on their health. He also observed that the Inuit obtained all the vitamins they needed from their traditional winter diet, even though this contained no plant matter; vitamin C, for example, was found in raw meat such as ringed seal liver and whale skin (Fediuk 2000, 5–6, 95). Another aspect of Inuit life worth stressing relates to the domestication of animals. They relied on dogs which had been tamed and bred from wild wolf stock, and these huskies would protect the camp from bears, serve as pack animals, pull sledges across ice and snow and accompany the men on hunting expeditions.

Sami

On the extreme northern margins of Europe reindeer hunters are still found. A pack of wolves would often accompany wild reindeer on their move from summer to winter pastures, picking off the stragglers (the very young or very old) on their migration, while leaving a fully viable core of the herd intact. The Sami of northern Norway (Europe's last surviving indigenous people) perhaps once followed and hunted reindeer in much the same symbiotic way, but they then learned to intercept the animals at a particular point on the seasonal migration, before subsequently herding and culling the deer, while still driving them from summer to winter pastures. A separate population, the sea Sami, settled on the coast and took up intensive fishing with some localised small farming. Thus the same indigenous people developed two quite contrasting survival strategies in this demanding environment.

Yanomamo

Another tribe who arguably lived on the cusp of the Neolithic Revolution in splendid isolation from the modern world until the 1960s, were the 20,000 people of the Yanomamo who were studied by Napoleon Chagnon (1997), among others. They were dispersed across the tropical forests that border Brazil and Venezuela, living in communities of 80 to 100 souls. Some of the smallest groups lived a very migratory life, making best use of the seasonal abundance of plant and animal foods in what archaeologists would regard as 'classic' hunter-gatherer mode. The majority, however, had settled in relatively permanent villages around which were clearings in the forest forming small fields or gardens. Although requiring considerable effort not just to clear the sites but also to tend and cultivate them successfully, these 'gardens' produced crops such as plantains in sufficient quantity to form some 80% of their diet. In other words, some of the community had developed a form of subsistence agriculture/horticulture that was effective enough to provide a reliable staple. The work was demanding, but the product seems to have provided a more consistent return for a rather larger group than a less sedentary hunter-gatherer group could anticipate. The diet of plantain was augmented by game hunted locally and by the collection of wild vegetable foods from the forest, ranging from various palm fruits, such as kareshi and vei, brazil nuts, tubers, seeds, pods, mushrooms and feral 'bananas'.

That said, the comforts of the home village – with its ready supply of food nearby – notwithstanding, the urge to go hunting for extended periods of time remained strong: old habits die hard. These episodes of 'camping' involved groups of up to 40 people living directly off the uncultivated lands. The sites were carefully selected to take maximum advantage of areas where ripening fruits would be in season and where game could be readily antici- pated. Even then, the family would take at least modest quantities of garden-grown plantain with them to ensure no one would go hungry (Chagnon 1997, 60). Once the seasonal fruits had been exhausted, the group would return to their home village and garden culture once again.

Trobrianders

Another community which cultivated gardens were the Trobrianders of Papua New Guinea. Although famous in anthropological circles for their journeys between the islands of the Massim as the 'Argonauts of the Western Pacific', it is their terrestrial adventures that will be reported on here. The islanders grow sweet potatoes, tapioca root, green beans, squash, bananas and bread fruit, items that presumably were once gathered directly in the wild. But they also grow yams, and these have become so important to their culture that the months of the year are named to reflect each stage of growth. Once harvested, the yams are stored in special huts and a period of *mwasawa* is declared between July and September, after which the labori- ous work starts on preparing the gardens for the next crop. Sometimes there is a formal competition to see who can produce the most, with the winners being rewarded with stone axes or similar valued items.

Kuvi yams can grow up to 6 feet in length or up to 2 feet in diameter and are far more than mere food: they are a sign of wealth and status for the gardener, the chief and the village. During the *mwasawa* festival, young peo- ple from 20 or 30 surrounding villages come together to celebrate the harvest with dancing and singing and much else besides. They even indulge in 'cricket' matches, but not with any rules that Lord's would recognise, since there are up to 50 people in a team. The initial impetus for this initiative came from local missionaries, who introduced the sport as a substitute for the sometimes inevitable inter-village fighting (Weiner 1988, 111–116). Much of the social, economic, political and cultural life of the community therefore revolves around this crop – perhaps an insight into life during the early Neolithic period.

It should be stressed that no modern-day indigenous tribe is likely to be conducting its affairs in exactly the same way as its ancestors would have done half a million years before; substantial changes would inevitably have been made over that long period, as the above examples show. Nonetheless, some of the basic societal, dietary and physical elements of our own prehistoric ancestry must be at least partially reflected in these mirrors, as is the diversity, resourcefulness and adaptability of such communities. In addition, modern archaeological research from across the globe has refined, dated and expanded our views of Stone Age society, physiology, nutrition and activity regimes, as the studies summarised in Chapters 4 to 7 show.

It seems that our lifestyles have now changed out of all recognition, as dramatically as the world's population has exploded. Those of us living in technologically driven towns might justifiably think that our Palaeolithic past has been left far behind. Although such studies certainly tell us something about a shared pre-urban past, is it any more than the stuff of academic debate? This book suggests that our bodies, and even part of our minds, retain an active ancestral legacy from distant – or not so distant – eras that still impacts directly upon us. Our uncivilised past is many, many millennia longer than the history of our civilisations.

Authorised version?

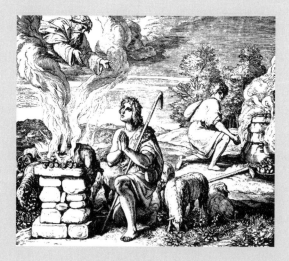

Clash of agricultures: Abel, the shepherd, attracts the malevolent attentions of Cain, the cereal killer.

The Old Testament comprises a collection of stories gathered together from a long oral tradition. Given that they were not written down until about 1000 BC, they must represent events, half-forgotten histories or much embellished tales from an even earlier era. Although these earlier entries may not be literally 'true', they may nonetheless be a symbolic version of genuine events. What follows is how an archaeologist might interpret part of the Genesis story, taking into account what we now know about the sequence of human social and economic development in that part of the ancient world. As such, it arguably provides a more poetic perspective on the seismic event that saw *Homo sapiens* abandon the long established foraging regime for a brave new world of farming and urbanisation, summarised in this table into five phases:

Archaeological chronology	Genesis chronology
Phase 1: Hunter-gatherers Foraging, scavenging and hunting were the principal survival modes for our ancestors for most of our long prehistory.	**Phase 1: Hunter-gatherers** Garden of Eden: Adam and Eve represent hunter-gathering foragers in a land of plenty, until they are expelled.
Phase 2: Neolithic Revolution Old regimes began disappearing with the advent of intensive animal husbandry (domestication of animals, e.g. sheep and cows) and widespread growing of cereal crops (domestication of plants). Crops could be grown in quantity and to order in fixed, irrigated, cultivated fields; yields might therefore increase tenfold.	**Phase 2: Neolithic Revolution** The Tree of Knowledge provided an understanding of how plants and animals developed, and therefore how the natural world could be manipulated for human advantage. Adam and Eve's offspring were Cain "a tiller of the ground" (domestication of plants) and Abel "a keeper of sheep" (domestication of animals).
Phase 3: Territorial conflict The new regimes were capable of supporting much larger populations, but necessitated laying out boundaries, territories and fixed field systems where once the land had been open. As populations grew, this would lead to disputes over territory and resources.	**Phase 3: Territorial conflict** The disputes this revolution brought with it (e.g. herds trampling and eating fields of sown crops) are perhaps recalled in the infamous murder of Abel by his brother, Cain.
Phase 4: Urbanisation Larger population densities led to the growth of more permanent settlements, towns and cities, developing marketplaces for exchange of surplus agricultural products etc.	**Phase 4: Urbanisation** Cain's crop-growing dynasty flourished once he had moved to new lands where "he builded a city", named after his son, Enoch.

Archaeological chronology	Genesis chronology
Phase 5: Bronze and Iron Age The new agricultural regimes meant that food production was no longer the key daily imperative for all the population, so towns could now support the development of new occupations, specialisms and technologies, such as metalworking.	**Phase 5: Bronze and Iron Age** Enoch's great-great grandson Lamech "took two wives: Adah and Zillah". Their offspring included, "Jabal, the father of such as dwell in tents, and have cattle … Jubal, the father of all such as handle the harp and organ, and Tubal-Cain, an instructor of every artificer in brass and iron". Thus on the back of the successful arable farmers arose towns, providing a market focus for nomadic animal herders, for music and culture, as well as for the new bronze and iron technologies and culture.

The Genesis story might therefore reflect a misremembered memory of a long-gone era when Eden's foragers relied on the certainties of nature's bounty for survival: the expulsion was still recalled as a traumatic event which saw nature replaced by the uncertainties of farming and depending on their own resources. Some would argue that the loss of innocence has still not been fully resolved to this day (e.g. Berman 2000). Whatever the truth of the matter, it seems that it was revered as a cataclysmic event of such profound significance that it survived telling and retelling for several thousand years. If so, it's a distant memory of our evolutionary origins that has stayed with us, as indeed has our Palaeolithic genome.

In reality, we are still dealing with the fallout from those ancient agricultural and urban revolutions. It is relatively easy to prove that our physiology has still not fully adapted to those changes; we can also suggest that our minds are still deeply locked in the mindset of a Stone Age hunter-gatherer culture. We simply have not had sufficient evolutionary time to catch up. Genetically, we have the body and the spirit of Stone Age hunter-gatherers, shoehorned into 21st-century civilisations. This could be a cause of inner conflict for us as individuals and for society as a whole. We can, however, promote ways to adapt to modern society by making better use of our Palaeolithic past, in recognition of the long, long time we spent in that mythical garden.

Genetically speaking, it's not our original sin we need to address, but our original biology.

Chapter 4

A HUNGER GAME

Food first, then morality.

Bertolt Brecht (1898–1956)

Survival rations

It's hard for modern urbanised societies to appreciate food: it's taken for granted that there will be enough, and if one supermarket runs out of sun-dried tomatoes, then the one further down the road may well have them. Shopping for food is now a small part of the daily round, something done on the way home from work or left until the weekend to get everything in one go. Life wasn't always like that: for hunter-gatherer communities, collecting their food was not seen as a largely inconsequential but necessary inconvenience, it was a central focus: food was everything. The whole daily schedule was based around it, going out to find it, hunting or collecting it, then carrying it back to the settlement to prepare and finally eat it. Each day, every day, enough food had to be found from somewhere. Living off the land is demanding when little can be taken for granted, especially when the resources change with the seasons (what would we do if all our supermarkets closed for six months of the year?). For our ancestors, the need to eat was programmed into their survival kit: feeling hungry wasn't a state of mind, it was a call to action.

How things have changed. Today, while some benighted nations slowly starve, obese urban nations sit upon agricultural surpluses. Where is the middle ground in these hunger games? That is a far bigger question than this book can begin to address; nevertheless, a crucial starting point can be suggested. A human evolutionary perspective on our nutritional needs can help us to identify what we should not be eating, what we should be eating, how much of it we should be eating and why we should be eating it. This chapter tries to answer these fundamental questions, what our ancestral nutritional regimes comprised of and how they often differ from their modern counterparts.

Letters on corpulence

Links have long been made between diet, obesity and 'good health', as the remarkable case of William Banting (1797–1878) demonstrates. He was a London undertaker just 5 foot, 5 inches (1.65 m) tall but seriously over-weight. Since he was very worried by this, he had taken up rowing on the Thames every morning. Through this increased activity he recorded that he "gained muscular vigour, but with it a prodigious appetite", which he felt compelled to indulge. He discussed this conundrum with a friendly surgeon who advised him to "forsake the exercise". So much for professional medical advice. Ironically, that friend died shortly afterwards and Banting was obliged to seek help elsewhere (Lindeberg 2010, 132).

By the time he was 65, he weighed over 14 stone (around 91.7 kg), he had a body mass index (BMI) of 33.6 (calculated by dividing weight in kg by height in m^2) and he was suffering from diabetes, slow healing abscesses, reduced vision and impaired hearing, and so consulted the ear surgeon William Harvey. That gentleman was familiar with the publications of a French food writer, Jean Anthelme Brillat-Savarin, in particular his *The Physiology of Taste*, published in 1825 (see http://www.gutenberg.org/etext/5434), which suggested that high starch foods were a major cause of obesity (Lindeberg 2010, 27). Consequently, Harvey recommended a change in diet for Banting which, after only six months, improved his hearing and sight and dramatically reduced his BMI to 25. The permitted foods in the miracle diet were meat or fish every day, a little fruit and plenty of vegetables. The new regime was rich in protein, low in fat and had a low glycaemic load. Bread, butter, milk, sugar, beer and potatoes were excluded, all items which had "for many years been adopted freely" by the patient. Banting was surprised that his weight loss was achieved by exchanging a meagre diet for a more generous one, but confidently stated in his *Letters on Corpulence* (1863) that "the *quantity* of diet may be safely left to the natural appetite, and that it is the *quality* only which is essential to abate and cure corpulence" (see Lindeberg 2010, 132–133, italics in original).

Anatomical determinants of diet

Banting correctly identified that the quality of food in a diet was crucial to its success, but why were particular foods 'good' for you and others 'bad' for you? The answer requires a change to the actual question since it is not the fault of the foods themselves, but lies deep in the evolutionary history of the creature itself. When considering appropriate diets for particular mammals, the first factor to study is the jaw, together with the shape, size and number of teeth. A look into our modern mouths shows that we have incisors and canines, useful for cutting and shearing meat (imagine that task before the invention of knives and forks). We also have premolars for chewing plant matter and molars for crunching and grinding harder elements such as nuts. The human jaw is therefore a useful toolkit for an unspecialised omnivore, rendering them capable of dealing with a wide range of potential food sources (and thus surviving in a wide range of environments).

Next there is the digestive system, which for us and for all other creatures evolved and mutated over many generations in response to the food resources that were most regularly exploited. As with the teeth, so with the stomach: that of a herbivore differs from that of a fruit-eater, or from insectivores, carnivores or omnivores, such as humans or pigs. Apes and humans share many basic features of gut anatomy and digestive kinetics, reflecting their common ancestry. We both have a simple acid stomach, a small intestine, small cecum with an appendix and a sacculated colon. But there are differences reflecting different dietary regimes. In humans, 56% of gut volume is in the small intestine, whereas in apes it is the colon which is relatively larger. This relates directly to their need to accommodate a lower quality diet of bulky plant matter, whereas in humans our small intestine is better adapted to a nutritionally dense and more digestible diet than an ape would enjoy (Milton 1999b).

Clearly, different mammals are better equipped to consume different diets. Even the term 'omnivore' is not what it seems, for humans, although classified as omnivores, cannot sensibly or safely digest literally anything. They can, however, benefit from a wide variety of nutrients, basically the standard range of food types that must have been more or less available during the extended period of our hunter-gatherer evolution. The list is long and includes fresh vegetables, fruits, berries, nuts, roots, bulbs, non-grass seeds, larvae, insects, sundry animals (both muscle meat and all the innards), birds, eggs, fish and shellfish. These are the 'normal' foods that our bodies can readily convert into energy or into developing a strong, growing skeleton (Lindeberg 2010, 30–34). And then there are over-processed foods and sundry additives that are alien to our bodies, items that our stomachs or livers find harder to process or, indeed, can find no sensible use for. Such abnormal foods impact adversely on our physiology and our wellbeing, as William Banting discovered to his cost. It is of obvious importance that we all have a clear understanding of which fuels work for us (i.e. the foods that our evolving digestive systems can deal with efficiently), as opposed to the ones that provide little in the way of nutrients, have harmful side effects or that are no more than slow poisons. Nutritional science needs a full appreciation of the evolutionary rationale that underpins our wellbeing.

We are what we ate

It can therefore be accepted that the environmental niches that herbivores, carnivores and omnivores inhabit are reflected in their different physiologies and digestive systems, and ultimately in the range of foods that they are best adapted to collect and consume. For humans, this complex balance of physiology and the associated preferred nutritional regimes is embedded in our genome. It was not implanted there as a fixed entity seven million years ago, but developed over time and many, many generations. It is thus largely a product moulded by the dictates of undirected natural selection, that mechanistic process which only ensures the survival of the fittest. As a consequence, it provides us with a very tried and tested model of a digestive system that is efficient enough and adaptable enough to cope with living in the wild from the equator to the Arctic Circle. It was and is capable of supporting a lifestyle broadly free from obesity, cardiovascular problems and diabetes, but only on its own terms.

Put simply, our bodies cannot cope with a diet that diverges drastically from those basic evolutionary-concordant rules, since that leads directly to today's apparently unstoppable rise in western lifestyle diseases. We need to identify precisely what we used to gather, hunt and eat in the long era before urbanisation, and rediscover what works best for our biology. To repeat, it's not that there are 'good' and 'bad' foods; it's just that some are compatible with our uncivilised genes and some are decidedly not. Fortunately, archaeological and anthropological evidence is already clarifying and expanding our knowledge of the dietary regimes adopted by our hunter-gatherer ancestors in the differing environments they successfully exploited (e.g. Brothwell and Brothwell 1998; Stanford and Bunn 2001; Ungar 2006; Kiple and Kriemhild 2012). We can no longer plead ignorance. Foods (or additives) that have been part of the human staple diet for less than 10,000 years have not been as rigorously tested by natural selection. As Staffan Lindeberg says, "Dietary advice to prevent and treat common Western diseases should be designed in accordance with our human biological heritage" (Lindeberg 2010, 29).

Food from the forest: first fruits

The story is a long one, but we will start somewhere in the middle, with the physiology of the direct ancestors of the human race. As they evolved, so too did the generalities of their associated diets: some 20 million years ago, a species of fruit-eating, four-footed climbing ape called Proconsul lived in the tropical forests of Africa. Echoes of these ancient frugivores still survive in our digestive system and also in our palate: our modern-day love of sugar dates back to an age when fruit was ripe enough to eat only when it tasted sweet. An interesting example of a modern mammal with a decided preference for small ripe fruits is the owl monkey, often found foraging in the crowns of tropical forest trees where such fruits grow all year round. However, in dry forest conditions, seasonality comes into play, obliging the owl monkeys in these regions to eat far more leaves, flowers and even insects.

A similar adaption seems to have occurred some ten million years ago in our own long ancestry when two quite distinct lineages appear in the evolving ape fossil record. The remains of one group, *Ankarapithecus meteai*, has been found in regions that were either non-tropical or highly seasonal, and seem to show anatomical adaptions for locomotion on the ground as well as in trees. An environment with less dense tree cover than a tropical forest would also provide different potential food resources, and it is significant to record that the apes here had large teeth, with thick enamel, set in robust jaws. This suggests that, rather than just soft tropical fruits, harder items such as nuts, woody fruits and seeds could be consumed. Thus, as these Miocene apes began exploiting the more open regions or woodlands beyond the tropical forests, the offspring of those who were better suited anatomically to these different environments multiplied, with sundry adaptions and mutations.

Precisely what happened next is still the subject of research, but some six million years ago there was a clear divergence in the lineage of the ape-like creatures, with one branch ultimately represented by chimpanzees and another represented by early hominins. A fundamental dietary change for hominins has also been demonstrated by isotopic analysis of the teeth of ancient primates. Evidence for the foods we once ate and the environments from which they were derived is recorded in the isotopic signatures left in our bones and teeth. Leaves, soft shoots, green stems and fruits are classified as C3 foods, and these can be identified by the distinctive isotopic traces left in the tooth enamel of browsers living in or close to well-wooded environments. A different chemical signature identifies C4 food types, which is characteristic of grazers feeding on ground level vegetation, such as grasses or tubers. A recent study by Professor Naomi Levin's team from Johns Hopkins University, Baltimore, analysed 152 fossil teeth from early humans and other ancient mammals from sites in Africa. The earlier mammals were predominantly C3 browsers, but then there was a significant change. There is clear evidence from the teeth of human-like species such as *Australopithecus afarensis*, *Australopithecus africanus* and *Kenyanthropus platyops*, which lived between 3.9 million and 2 million years ago, that they had also absorbed C4 plant matter (Levin et al. 2015). This certainly reflects a major ecological change to be adapted to, with the apparent increased development of open grassland rather than dense tree cover. It also shows that our early ancestors were consequently widening their dietary regime beyond the familiar fruits of the forest. It now began to include wild grasses, either directly or, as Professor Robert Tykot comments, "indirectly through herbivorous faunal intermediaries" (Tykot 2004, 436), which translates as "eating the animals that were eating the grass".

Fresh water

The central importance of simple water in our nutritional regimes is often overlooked, at least in urbanised western cultures. It was not always thus. Indeed, as Christianity slowly tried to impose its monotheistic values on the largely pagan population of these isles, the worship of water at wells or springs were alternative practices that proved very hard to eradicate. In the eighth century AD, Egbert's Penitential decried the making of offerings at wells, while the early 11th-century Canons of Edgar forbade the worship of wells and similar heathen activities (Morris 1989, 60). The laws of King Cnut (c.1020) defined pagan practice as the worship of things like trees or wells (Whitelock 1979, 455), while contemporary Northumbrian Priests' Law summarised the punishments to be meted out for those with sanctuaries focused on stones, trees, wells "or other such nonsense" (Whitelock 1979, 475). Well-worship is therefore mentioned in very different sources over a wide date range and continuing for several hundred years after the introduction of Christianity by the Augustine mission in AD 597.

This suggests that an ancient reverence for water was once commonplace and deeply felt. In some areas, Christianity only triumphed over the water gods by quite literally subsuming them: there are many examples of churches built directly over wells, such as St Peter's, Barton-upon-Humber, which has three wells at its east end (Rodwell and Rodwell 1982, 293, fig. 6), St Helen-on-the-Walls, York, where the chancel was extended over a well (Magilton 1980, 17, fig. 5a), and the Old Minster in Winchester, which had been built over and around a number of wells (Biddle 1970, fig. 12). In London, a well seems to have been the focus for the 11th-century church of St Bride's, and a series of them continued to be recut and used until the early 19th century: the area around the church is still known as Bridewell (Milne 1997, 110–111).

Water may no longer be worshipped, but it is now most certainly valued, since premium prices are paid for the 'pure' product. As for humble tap water, a cheaper option, that too has its supporters: some suggest it should be taken hot or warm first thing in the morning, while others recommend it cold as an excellent accompaniment for meals (e.g. Lindeberg 2010, 228).

Food from the field: ancestral nutritional regimes

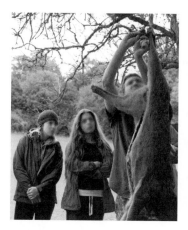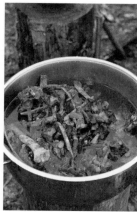

Figure 4.1. Carnivores: once killed, animals were skinned (left), cut up and cooked; even bones provide nourishment (right).

The next significant evolutionary anatomical change sees the gradual selection of the characteristic features now seen as representing *Homo erectus*, or *Homo ergaster*, from about 1.8 million years ago. This species had a larger brain than its immediate predecessor (*Homo habilis*) implying greater cognitive abilities and perhaps a greater ability to respond to change. Of particular relevance to this chapter, these ancestors also had a smaller gut and smaller molar teeth. This suggests less reliance on raw plant food in the diet, since many plants need to be chewed repeatedly and need time to digest thoroughly (Stringer and Andrews 2011, 204–206). This raises an important question: does a change in the dietary regime suggest changes in the environment and resources available, or just changes in the physiology of the consumers, or were both adapting to each other (Ungar 2006)?

The body requires energy to run all its organs, and the amount of energy can be quantified through calculations related to the basal metabolic rate. According to a pioneering paper published some 20 years ago (Aiello and Wheeler 1995; see also Milton 1999b), the increase in human brain size at the same time as the decrease in gut size are related: such a change would suggest a higher quality diet was being obtained, and this may have involved more meat, rather than an increased amount of plant-based foods. Cows need seven stomachs to digest their grassy diet; modern humans have just the one internal stomach. But then an external stomach was invented, following the domestication of fire. The invention of cooking provided us with semi-digested food. Cooking makes substances like starches more digestible and also neutralises toxins; cooked food is therefore easier and quicker for the body to convert into nutrients and energy than the raw components themselves. Eating substantial amounts of animal-derived cooked food is a very cost-effective way of obtaining valuable protein when compared with the energy required to obtain a similar scale of benefit from raw plant foods. Although the evolving bipedal upright creatures supported a relatively small gut, the ingestion of more long-chain fatty acids, which are far more plentiful in meats, provided more energy to develop the brain.

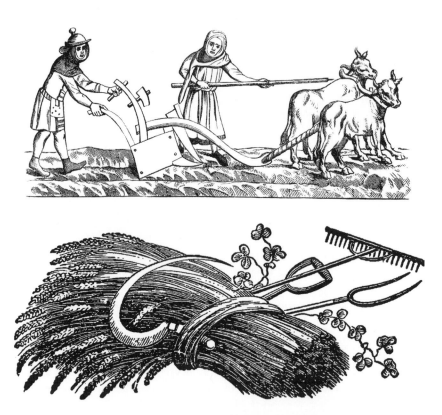

Figure 4.2. Domestication of plants: growing cereals extensively required open fields and considerable labour, as well as a range of new tools and equipment from ploughs (top) to sickles (bottom).

An implication of these marked changes in physique and metabolism is that these early humans, rather than being reactive, opportunistic meat-eaters who sought out the carcasses of creatures that had already died or been killed by other predators, were now increasingly well-adapted as proactive hunters. Some support for this suggestion comes from the increasing use of stone tools such as bifaces or hand axes, carefully shaped with edges designed to cut up and skin carcasses quickly and effectively. The speedy processing of prey at a kill site is an imperative, since other predators – be they vultures, hyenas or lions – would all be keen to take a share. Thus, the development of proactive hunting skills, the ability to process animal carcasses and, finally, the means to cook meat may all have played their part in bringing about this gradual but profound physiological and social change (see e.g. Stanford 1999; Stanford and Bunn 2001). It seems that, by this period, our ancestors were no longer frugivores, but had developed a physiology, a culture and a taste for meat, although vegetables remained firmly on the menu (Hardy et al. 2015).

It is self-evident that the environmental niches that herbivores, frugivores, carnivores and omnivores inhabit are reflected in their different physiologies and digestive systems and in the foods they are specifically adapted to collect and consume. Archaeological evidence has clarified and expanded our knowledge of the varied dietary regimes developed by our own ancestors. This widening database has been compared and illuminated by anthropological research over the last century or so, with the study of communities that continued with their ancestral lifestyles well into the age of advancing modernity (e.g. Brothwell and Brothwell 1998; Stanford and Bunn 2001; Ungar 2006; Cohen 2012; Kiple and Kriemhild 2012; Wing 2012).

At the head of this chapter, the dietary regime of William Banting was described: it was a proxy 'ancestral diet' in all but name and origin. One of the first major scientific studies that made deliberate conscious links between ancestral diets, primitive physiology and modern man was published in 1939. It was written by Weston Price, a distinguished North American dentist who compared the teeth, dental-arch and facial deformities observed in those eating a modern 'westernised' diet with those who preferred a traditional 'native' diet. His focus rested on the societies more or less untouched by 'civilisation' or urbanisation that produced seemingly healthy people (although he was acutely aware of other tribes that were surviving far less successfully into the 20th century). His book, with its detailed text and copious illustrations, bore the title *Nutrition and Physical Degeneration: A Comparison of the Primitive and Modern Diet and Their Effects.*

Although the central focus was on dentition and dental diseases, it ranged over other related issues, and was arguably one of the first major scientifically compiled studies to advocate the positive health benefits of a 'native' or ancestral diet over a modern one. Not only did he record fine teeth, but he also noted the marked absence of tuberculosis, arthritis, heart disease and other conditions rather too familiar to modern society. The dietary research encompassed 'primitive' communities right across the globe. Some of these isolated societies included smallholders with modest allotments and some livestock, while others could be classified as hunter-gatherer. The first category included the Gaelic-speaking crofters on the Inner and Outer Hebridean islands off Scotland. They harvested the sea for fish and crustaceans, but also grew such vegetables as they could as well as oats for the staple porridge and oat cakes. Price also studied the dairy farmers of Löetschental high in the Swiss Alps, who lived on cheese, fresh vegetables, a little meat and rye bread.

From the second category, there were the Inuit of Alaska (sea mammals, fish and caribou); Native Americans living in the Rocky Mountains (moose, caribou and plants in the summer); Australian Aborigines (sundry plants, sea foods and wild animals); the New Zealand Maori (fruit, vegetables, birds and seafood) as well as Melanesians and Polynesians on eight archipelagos of the Southern Pacific (fish, shellfish, fruit and tubers). He also considered the diets of African tribes that varied according to the terrain: some hunted wild animals, others kept cattle and goats for meat and dairy, those that lived near freshwater lakes exploited the fish, but all enjoyed insects. All in all, he found a great dietary variety of game, seafood, fruit, vegetables, grain and dairy, all of which seemed to provide the consumers with strong bones, good teeth and a high immunity to dental caries, together with an absence from several other degenerative processes (Price 1939, ch. 15). Significantly, Price also recorded the negative effects inflicted upon those communities, their general health and their dentition when they adopted a more 'modern' lifestyle. He commented on this impact from tribes in Alaska, Kenya and the Torres Strait Islands, but also noted that when his colleague Dr Josef Romig prescribed a return to their traditional diets, many of the problems were subsequently resolved.

Further important insights have been gained working with evidence collated from the observation of an even wider range of hunter-gatherer populations that survived into the 20th century and into the age of anthropological study, as a recent study of 229 examples shows (Cordain et al. 2000). First of all there was no strict single 'ancestral diet' shared by all the groups, since the regimes were operating across the globe in very contrasting environments. But all were nutrient rich, and all included the fat-soluble vitamins A, D and E as well as K, so often missing from modern menus (Minger 2013, 236). Taken as a whole, the species eaten varied dramatically from country to country, and so too did the ratio of plant-based foods to meat and fish. The proportion of the hunter-gatherer diets that relied upon gathered plant foods varied from 26% to 35%, and a similar figure and similar range were recorded for hunted animals and fished foods. In other words, a 'standard ancestral diet' (if there was one) might have comprised one-third plants, one-third animals, one-third fish. That said, the ratio changed dramatically with latitude: the closer the groups were to the Arctic Circle, the percentage of animals vis-à-vis the plant foods became greater as the vegetation became sparser in the regions they inhabited.

Of all the 229 ancestral diets listed, however, none were based solely on plant matter: all had at least some meat included. There were, apparently, no vegetarians or vegans in those particular worlds; indeed, 46 of the communities catalogued were highly or solely dependent on hunted, trapped or fished creatures. Of five African communities studied for which quantitative data are available, it seems that meat/fish constituted 26%, 33%, 44%, 48% and 68% of the food supply. Once again, there was no one uniform 'ancestral diet', although they share clear commonalities – for example, the macronutrient consumption ratios for many hunter-gatherer populations seemed to have favoured protein over carbohydrate. Seasonality and altitude also played major roles in determining what and when resources were available, and for how long; in other words, adaptability and flexibility were key (Cordain et al. 2000). (The catch-all term hunter-gatherer also includes gatherer-hunters, hunter-fishers and fisher-gatherers – see Appendix 1, 'Hunter-gatherers with latitude'.)

The list of foods that were consumed is long and includes sundry plants, nuts, insects, large and small animals, birds and fish. To that menu can also be added the 'underground storage organs' such as roots, tubers and bulbs (Laden and Wrangham 2005). Given the environments that *Homo sapiens* and their immediate ancestors are known to have colonised, such fare could have been available and exploited for millennia, as suggested by archaeological research. In terms of our Palaeolithic genome, these are seen as the foods the human digestive system is most adept at processing efficiently: fresh foods, in a great variety of forms and thus a great variety of micronutrients as well. A detailed study of the plant foods utilised by Australian Aborigines demonstrates this variety: dictated by changing locations and changing seasons, 41% were fruits, 26% seeds or nuts, and 24% tubers and roots, with leaves, flowers and other plant parts making up the remaining 9%. There was not a monotonous or reliable daily staple in sight. It is clear that, while dairy and grain products can be consumed by some without detriment, neither seem to be essential or universal mainstays of the optimal diet. Which brings us, on cue, to the Neolithic Revolution.

Food from the farm: Neolithic nutritional regimes

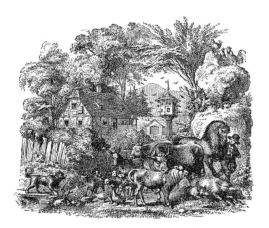 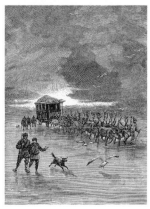

Figure 4.3. The domestication of animals was not just for food, but also for milk and skins (left) and as beasts of burden (right).

'Good health' is fuelled by a dietary regime that our ancient digestive system and metabolism consider 'normal' (i.e. to which our biology has had enough time to adapt). So what happened as a consequence of the changes introduced during the Neolithic period? The advent of cereal farming and animal husbandry brought 'new' foods to the table in quantity, if not in quality: grass seeds from the Poaceae family, although they do not seem to have featured directly in ancestral human diets, now took centre stage – for example, wheat, barley, oats, rye, maize and rice. Meat from domesticated animals (rather than lean game from the wild) as well as milk and other dairy products were also introduced, again items that were formerly alien to the human palate and digestive system.

Evidence from 11,000 BP suggests that new, more intensive agricultural regimes originated in the Fertile Crescent (in modern-day Iraq). Much larger populations from a relatively compact territory could be supported by cereal cultivation, given reliable harvests. The new approaches soon spread to the Jordan Valley, by which date sheep, goats, cows and pigs had all been domesticated (or at least semi-domesticated) to provide another controlled and reliable source of food. Across the globe it seems that similar practices developed quite independently. Rice, cultivated in irrigated fields, became the new staple in China, initially in the Yangtze and Yellow River basins, by at least 9,000 BP. In the New Guinea Highlands, between 9,000 and 6,000 BP, the focus was on bananas and plantains, while the earliest such agricultural developments from eastern sub-Saharan Africa date rather later to 5,000 and 4,000 BP, where a range of crops were husbanded, including millet and yams. On the other side of the world, in Central Mexico and northern South America, a variety of crops were grown extensively including maize in Mesoamerica and potatoes in South America. Thus across the globe, the human race summarily adopted and developed 'new' staples "for which the hominin genome had little evolutionary experience" (Cordain et al. 2005) and arguably is still playing catch-up.

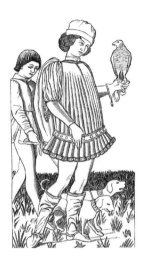

Figure 4.4. Domestication of birds: not just for meat, eggs and feathers but also as hunters.

For the new breed of farm labourers, shepherds and cowherds, much of their active daily lives were spent working in the fresh air, superficially an evolutionary-concordant activity regime. But archaeologists have compared the differences between the diet and physique of pre-agricultural foragers and the 'new' agriculturists. This was achieved by comparing the skeletal remains and other evidence of the two very contrasting groups. In the United States, for example, a detailed study by Kirstin Sobolik (University of Maine) of the coprolites (preserved faeces) left by foraging groups some 10,000 years ago – that is to say, before the 'new' agricultural practices became prevalent there – provides remarkably detailed information. It seems that the majority of the calories eaten by the foragers represented came from high-fibre plants such as the leaves of sotol and agave, from cactus pads, sunflower seeds, ground mesquite, acorns, walnuts and pecans, as well as from persimmons, grapes, blackberries and wild onions. The protein came from eating mice, pack rats, fish, freshwater clams, lizards, caterpillars, grasshoppers, birds and their eggs, rabbits and occasionally deer. Such wild animals as were eaten were lean creatures – quite unlike those bred for the table today – with less than 5% body fat. Such a wide-ranging diet represents a supremely adaptable, omnivorous approach to survival, eating whatever was in season, and shows a willingness to forage over a wide area in greatly differing environments, and thus accumulating greatly differing micronutrients (Sobolik 2012, 44–51). Karl Reinhard (University of Nebraska) has stressed the almost complete absence of evidence of debilitating intestinal parasites in these coprolites, in marked and striking contrast to the evidence recovered from the late agriculturalists. These later 'agricultural' groups showed clear evidence of anaemia and parasites such as tapeworms, pinworms and thorny-headed worms (Reinhard 2000; Reinhard and Bryant 2008; Reinhard et al. 2013).

The skeletal evidence gathered from studies of populations of prehistoric foragers and later agriculturalists is just as revealing, as Professor Armelagos (Emory University) has shown (Armelagos 1990). In the region around the Ohio and Illinois Valley, anaemia became a major problem after the advent of farming, when the American Indians began to rely heavily on maize as their primary staple, with little meat. Long-term debilitating iron deficiency seems to have been the cause of high levels of bone porosity, a condition known as porotic hyperostosis, which left its indelible signature on the skulls of those early farmers. There were also skeletal and dental changes recorded following the development of early agriculture in Georgia (Larsen 1981).

Similar unwelcome Neolithic developments have been identified in a major study involving 34,000 human skeletons excavated from British sites dating from 10,000 BC to the early modern period (Roberts and Cox 2003). The available prehistoric data suggested that although there was some evidence for dental caries and other dental defects in the Palaeolithic and Mesolithic period, there was a marked increase in these conditions in the Neolithic period. That era also saw the introduction of new features such as anaemia, osteoporosis, osteochondritis dissecans and diffuse idiopathic skeletal hyperostosis (DISH), which is associated with obesity. There were also new infections such as osteitis and periostitis of sinuses, ribs and skull (possible meningitis) and evidence of tumours.

Damning archaeological studies such as these have therefore shown that, while the new agriculturalists may have provided sufficient food to support a larger population, it was not necessarily a healthier or happier one. It seems the provision of heavyweight cereal staples effectively displaced much of the variety of pre-agricultural diets and, significantly, the associated micronutrients so important for our general health and for robust immune systems. Then there is the potential problem posed by alpha-amylase, the enzyme in our saliva that breaks down starch into useable sugars. Not all humans have the same number of AMY1 copies in their genetic make-up, and thus not all humans cope with starch in the same way. The high amylase group (with anything from 6 to 15 inherited copies) can digest starch relatively easily and use it to meet their energy requirements. However, this is not at all the case for the low amylase group (below 6), who seem to be at a far greater risk of insulin resistance and diabetes; they should not, repeat not, be depending on a cereal staple. Our close relation, the bonobo, has only four copies of AMY1, while our closer relation, the chimpanzee, has but two, as befits their low-starch, fruit-rich regime. Interestingly, it seems that human populations with a long history of starchy food exploitation, such as the Japanese and the Hadza of Tanzania, tend to have more copies of AMY1 than low starch eating populations such as hunter-gatherers in the Congo rainforest or pastoralists from Siberia (Minger 2013, 205–210). The implication here is that natural selection has, over time, selectively eliminated those families that were genetically unsuited to the new regime.

As for the introduction of dairy products to the menu, that too is a mixed blessing. Products such as hard cheeses contain valuable vitamin K2, so critical for healthy hearts and strong skeletal growth, for example. But hunter-gatherers, ancient or modern, usually stop producing the enzyme lactase in their digestive systems once they have been weaned. As a consequence, they cannot metabolise lactose, and thus, as adults, avoid drinking animal milk, since their digestive systems reject it. However, some modern populations have a mutation on chromosome 2 which eliminates the shutdown in lactase production. They are thus able to consume fresh milk throughout their lives without difficulty. Today, such 'lactase persistence' ranges from as much as 95% in northern Europe, down to 29% for Sicily, to less than 10% in some African and Asian countries (NIDDK 2014).

It seems clear that the foci of these very specific genetic populations reflect the communities that moved from foraging to animal husbandry regimes several millennia ago. The identification of milk proteins found in ceramic vessels from Hungary and Romania, for example, provides evidence for dairying in those regions some 7,900 to 7,450 years ago. These practices were probably introduced by the Neolithic people sharing the Linearbandkeramik Culture, according to Professor Mark Thomas from University College London (UCL). He has shown that most of today's European lactase-persistent populations now carry the same variant of the 13,910*T gene. Rather than being drunk fresh, it seems that animal milk was initially fermented to make cheeses, butter or yoghurts. But milk drinking ultimately spread rapidly with the more widespread husbandry of cattle, with Neolithic farmers reaching England some 6,100 years ago and settling in north-western Spain around 4,500 years ago (Gerbault et al. 2013).

In northern Europe, in the latitudes where altitude, environment and the consequences of climate change were less benevolent than the lands to the south, dairy produce may have become a major factor in the battle to survive. The lack of viable alternative staples and, once again, natural selection, would weed out those intolerant families, generation by generation, until most of the survivors in the gene pool were of the lactase-persistence variety (Lindeberg 2010, 6).

But there are even deeper costs directly related to milk and cereal consumption. Autoimmune diseases result from the body's immune system attacking its own cells and tissues. During our long evolution, our immune systems gradually 'learned' to identify potentially harmful bacteria and viruses, and subsequently supress them, thus providing a 'natural immunity' should a later attack materialise. But sometimes our autoimmune system fails to correctly distinguish between its own proteins and foreign interlopers in 'new' foods consumed (i.e. foods that the digestive system had not previously experienced and thus had no familiarity with). Those new but unwelcome agents – items only introduced to the human body during the Neolithic Revolution – can then work their way through the intestinal wall, breached by lectins in cereal grains and beans (Lindeberg 2010, 210–212).

It is worth pausing here to consider the subject of epigenetics. The genome you inherited at birth is yours for life and yours to pass on to your children. The genes themselves are broadly stable and provide a picture of what could be termed your biological potential (for good or for ill). However, what actually happens to you depends to a certain extent on how those genes are expressed – that is, how they function or mis-function. You might have inherited a predisposition for, say, coronary heart disease, but that does not mean you will inevitably suffer from it. Epigenetics studies the processes that determine how and why certain genes are activated while others are suppressed during your lifetime. Such biological modifications are regular occurrences but can also be influenced, often markedly, by factors including age, lifestyle and the diseases you suffer from. These changes do not, as a rule, modify the genetic code sequence of your DNA. But your lifestyle choices can, in certain cases, modify the expression of those changes.

To take an example: there are plenty of individuals who can and do eat cereals without any immediately obvious major complications, beyond the fact that such staples when eaten in bulk have displaced more nutritious foods and micronutrients from the menu. But there are many for whom consuming the gluten from grains, such as modern strains of wheat and rye, promotes coeliac disease – the destruction of the intestinal mucosal membrane. This is but one form of gluten intolerance; an autoimmune skin disease called dermatitis herpetiformis is another, for example. Staffan Lindeberg records a number of studies concerning related conditions such as a motion coordination disorder, now called gluten ataxia, and a disease of the peripheral nervous system (peripheral neuropathy). He notes that, for some modern patients today, a gluten-free diet provides the simplest cure – that is to say, one that avoids the Neolithic Revolution (Lindeberg 2010, 212) and the debilitating conditions it can trigger.

Many patients with rheumatoid arthritis, especially those with the rheumatoid factor in their blood, display antibodies against wheat or milk proteins (Lindeberg 2010, 212–213). The distribution of type 1 diabetes, an autoimmune reaction that destroys insulin-producing cells in the pancreas, is strongly correlated with populations consuming dairy products (Lindeberg 2010, 213–214). So too is the geographical distribution of multiple sclerosis (MS), an autoimmune disease of the brain and spinal cord that is now an all too common occurrence in modern western societies: immunity against cow milk proteins and antibodies against wheat gluten have been found in many MS patients. Once again, a strong case can be made for the positive reintroduction of evolutionary-concordant dietary regimes (and the exclusion of cereal and dairy products) to address such serious issues in particular individuals (Lindeberg 2010, 214–215).

The archaeological evidence shows that the Neolithic period was one of long-term population expansion. The challenges posed by increased dependence on cereals (and therefore on abundant harvests), animal husbandry and dairy products were not, however, always successfully overcome, at least in the short term in Europe. Following the introduction of these innovative agricultural practices into south-eastern Europe 8,500 years ago and their subsequent spread throughout the continent, rather than sustaining a steady population growth what actually followed was an alarming boom-and-bust cycle in population densities. Initial suggestions indicate declines in the order of 30–60% in some instances, not dissimilar to the impact of the Black Death that struck Europe in the mid-14th century (Shennan et al. 2013).

The social and cultural implications of such changes must have been far reaching. The causes are unknown as yet, but in addition to possible plagues or other crowd infections, soil erosion, crop failures, animal or plant disease or warfare may all have had associated roles to play. It may be that the march of progress brought about by the Neolithic Revolution was accompanied not by diseases of affluence but by the diseases of agrarianism, 'the Neolithic Syndrome'. These were often conditions that, on their own would not necessarily be fatal. Nevertheless, it was a different matter for those weak or weakened sectors of the population who were genetically unsuited to dairy products or cereals, suffered from iron deficiency or whose immune systems felt the loss of the micronutrients enjoyed by hunter-gatherers, or were beset by a new wave of autoimmune diseases. Natural selection could not be argued with then.

Food from the factory: urbanised nutritional regimes

Life in towns in antiquity often did little to improve the situation, although much depended on the social stratum individuals were born into or found themselves thrown into. To take two ends of the spectrum: the domesticated, subjugated, servile or slave classes would have far less choice as to what they ate or in what quantity; for the ruling elites, on the other hand, the opposite situation presented itself, both in the range and amounts of food and drink that might be consumed. In the middle ground, however, it can be recorded that many of the smaller urban settlements often had fields and farms directly outside (or indeed inside) their city limits, and thus at least fresh fruit and vegetables could be procured without too much difficulty. Consequently, it is hard to define a common urban diet other than to note that people became ever more dependent on cereal-based staples which supplanted the rich variety of 'normal' ancestral regimes. As a result, the Neolithic Syndrome was never seriously addressed, and thus diseases and conditions related to dietary deficiencies in macro- and micronutrients persisted.

The osteological evidence archaeologically excavated from British sites is quite unequivocal, not to mention depressing (Roberts and Cox 2003; see also Appendix 2, 'Diseases of civilisation: osteological evidence from British cemetery excavations'): the prehistoric periods after the Neolithic (2600 BC– AD 50) saw further increases in metabolic, joint and dental disease as well as anaemia. It also saw the first evidence for spondylosis, some tumours and circulatory conditions such as Scheuermann's and Perthes' disease. Next, the introduction of fully formed towns following the Roman invasion of AD 43 was not entirely beneficial. The new civilisation introduced the first evidence of diet-related conditions such as scurvy, rickets, gout, osteomalacia and tapeworms, as well as another marked increase in anaemia and dental disease. The archaeological evidence for urban wellbeing in the Roman period is therefore somewhat mixed, as is the picture for later medieval urbanisation. From AD 1000 onwards there are further increases in the incidence of dental, congenital, neoplastic and metabolic diseases, DISH, Paget's disease, osteoporosis and gall stones. This period also saw the introduction and dramatic spread of bubonic plague, an infection that carried off millions, especially those whose bodies or immune systems had already been weakened by poor diet or famine.

What can also be shown is that as urban populations expanded with the Industrial Revolution the situation notably worsened. Food processing methodologies were increasingly developed to feed the urban masses, together with additives, preservatives and colourants. These were often at the expense of the nutritional and micro-nutritional value of the foods themselves. In addition, excessive amounts of sugar and imported products such as tobacco were introduced to the increasingly urbanised 'western' cultures. By over-processing and industrialising cereals, dairy and meat products, the

Neolithic Syndrome was exacerbated by over-indulgence and wide-ranging cultural changes, fuelling the rise of the 'diseases of affluence'. In the United States today, it has been calculated that dairy products, refined sugars, refined vegetable oils and alcohol comprise over 70% of the energy consumed by the population: it is sobering to learn that next to none of these types of food would have contributed to the energy component of any ancestral pre-agricultural diet. It should therefore come as no surprise that our biology is not coping too well with such abnormal fare.

We have already catalogued (see Chapter 1) the alarming list of diseases and conditions that have been labelled the 'diseases of affluence' or 'western lifestyle'. As for some of the potential causes and catalysts, evidence has been comprehensively published by others including Staffan Lindeberg (2010) to identify the prime suspects as far as modern urban diets are concerned. These studies show that, although our nutritional needs remain largely as they were three million years ago, modern urban diets have often moved too far away from such evolutionary-concordant regimes, resulting in an undue burden on our digestive systems, immune systems and consequently on the National Health Service. But the actual identification of the specific dietary elements that were most to blame for the poor health of modern urban populations has been a protracted and expensive criminal investigation, or rather, investigations. Was it dairy products, was it sugar, was it fat, was it cholesterol, was it meat, was it cereals? All these and more have come under the medical microscope over the last 70 years, with the results of individual studies being variously lauded or laughed at. Some of the more influential are summarised in the next chapter. At the same time, a growing interest in ancestral diets, not as an interesting sideline, but as a positive solution, has built and its once quiet voice now merits much wider attention.

Chapter 5

FOOD FOR THOUGHT

Man shall not live by bread alone.

Matthew 4:4

Health of nations

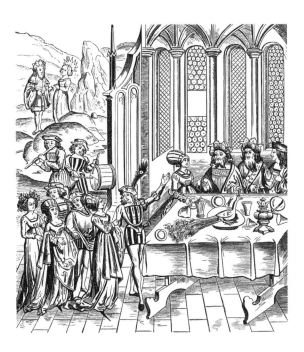

Figure 5.1. Table manners: medieval communal dining.

The Second World War inflicted unprecedented levels of destruction and death on whole nations: more civilians were killed or injured than those serving in the military in a period when the term 'non-combatant' lost its meaning. Mass starvation was used deliberately as a weapon against civilian populations whether in concentration camps or besieged or occupied towns. Although the mainland of Great Britain was not invaded, it was repeatedly bombed and the convoys importing supplies from overseas were mercilessly hunted by German U-boats. Food was in increasingly short supply, and thus had to be rationed.

In 1940, the British Ministry of Food set out the basic nutritional requirements for adults to stay 'fighting fit' during the course of the Second World
War (Patten 1985, 8). The basic weekly ration decreed by the government
was a practical compromise of nutritional and cultural requirements, tempered by the need to spread the pain more or less evenly across the
population. Home-produced fruit and vegetables in season were not
rationed, and thus provided the bulk of the diet, while meat was strictly
limited, with only 4 oz (100 g) of bacon and ham per week, for example.
This was not a dissimilar proportion of meat/vegetables to some ancestral
diets; indeed, the allocation has been described as a "virtual peasant diet"
(Zweiniger-Bargielowska 2000, 37). In war-time Britain, sugar was also in
short supply, and was restricted to a weekly ration of 8 oz (225 g), a major
factor in a pronounced fall in cases of dental caries and obesity. Dairy products such as milk (three pints or 1,800 ml), butter and cheese (both 2 oz or
50 g) were also rationed. Even tea, without which no English family could
be expected to live, was restricted to 2 oz (50 g) per person per week.
However, all children had daily doses of orange juice and cod-liver oil, while
those from the poorer families were provided with a free school meal
(Zweiniger-Bargielowska 2000, 31–45).

The rationing of sweets and sugar continued until 1953 and meat until July
1954. Thus for over ten years the population enjoyed a rather monotonous
but balanced diet comprising many vegetables and locally produced fruits,
but with far less meat, fat or sugar than would be deemed 'normal' today. In
terms of basic nutrition, while much of the world starved, the British population as a whole was arguably healthier than it had been in the 1930s and
obesity was not prevalent. The nationally imposed diet and the simultaneous
development of the new National Health Service saw levels of maternal and
infant mortality decline significantly, while the average age of death from
natural causes increased (the Luftwaffe excepted). Anthropometric data also
shows notable improvements in child health and physique: in addition to
improved diet, a vigorous activity regime was also in place. Severe petrol
shortages meant that walking to and from work or school became the norm,
for example (Zweiniger-Bargielowska 2000, 259–260).

It is accepted that there was no conscious relationship drawn by the Ministry
of Food between the ration book and ancestral diets. That said, the British
food rationing exercise could be regarded as a major intervention that tested
the value of elements of a broadly 'evolutionary-compliant' diet on an
entire nation. This is not, repeat not, an endorsement of world wars, but one
positive lesson that can be drawn from the nightmare is that where there is
real political will, real positive health benefits can ensue with remarkable
speed. Indeed, it shows that the dietary health of an entire urbanised nation
can be 'rewilded' within a generation: this was a public health intervention
on a truly national scale. But then it all went wrong.

Western lifestyle diseases: searching for public enemy number one

The post-war period in the West witnessed major expansion in food production and processing, coupled with a general consensus that more food – from whatever source – was the key to good living. This was an understandable reaction to the deprivations suffered by that generation, but did more food automatically equate with better health for the consumers? Not everyone agreed, and the sudden rise in heart disease related mortality troubled many. As a consequence, several major dietary and lifestyle studies were undertaken in an attempt to identify the causes of ill health in the modern world.

Saturated fat

One of these studies was undertaken by the nutritionist Ancel Keys (see Minger 2013, 89–103), the man who developed the K-rations for the American army during the war. He had noticed that heart disease related mortality had dropped rapidly in regions where systematic food rationing had been in place, when compared with areas in the industrialised world that had avoided such restrictions. He then studied 300 businessmen from upmarket Minnesota, looking for significant risk factors. This highlighted the men's total cholesterol levels, since there was a statistical association between those rising levels and the increasing likelihood of heart disease. This led to the next question: what caused those levels to rise? After further studies, Keys suggested that it was saturated fat that led to increased cholesterol levels, which led him to the suggestion that it was that which caused cardiovascular disease (see Minger 2013, 94–95).

The assumption that lay behind his diet–heart hypothesis was roundly condemned by some (Yerushalmy and Hilleboe 1957), but this did not prevent Keys from launching the major 'Seven Countries Study' of some 12,763 men (no women) aged between 40 and 59 living in villages in the United States, the Netherlands, Japan, Italy, Yugoslavia, Finland and Greece (Keys 1980). A systematic examination of these varied groups would look at the relationships between lifestyle, diet and coronary heart disease, with follow-up studies to track longer term results over the next 50 years. The first results broadly confirmed other contemporary studies undertaken in the United States – such as the Framingham Heart Study (Mahmood et al. 2014) – that had stressed the importance of not being overweight, taking regular exercise, eating a healthy diet and not smoking. It also suggested that the risk and rates of heart attack and stroke were related to higher levels of total serum cholesterol, and that cholesterol and obesity were associated with increased mortality from cancer. Again, it was suggested that dietary saturated fat seemed to be the masked killer. But was it as simple as that?

Sugar

Professor Yudkin disagreed, and took a different line, since he thought that sugar was the key culprit. He had founded the Department of Nutrition in London's Queen Elizabeth College in 1954, the first institution in Europe to award a BSc in nutrition. His own research was wide ranging, including work on adaptive enzymes, the social determinants of health and historical aspects of the human diet as well as public health issues and cultural dietary preferences. But the end of food rationing in the UK in the early 1950s brought with it an increase in the number of people who were suffering from obesity, and Yudkin showed that weight could be controlled by restricting dietary carbohydrate. This period also saw a rise in the incidence of coronary thrombosis, attributed by many to the amount of fat consumed. Yudkin, however, suspected that excessive sugar in the diet might be contributing not only to obesity but also to coronary heart disease. He found that increasing prosperity leads to an increase in sugar consumption, particularly in manufactured foods. In 1963 he wrote that in the wealthier countries, there is evidence that sugar and sugar-containing foods contribute to diseases such as obesity, dental caries, diabetes mellitus and heart attack, to which list he later added atherosclerotic disease (a frequent precursor of coronary heart disease), and subsequently gout, dyspepsia and some cancers. By 1967 he had suggested that excessive consumption of sugar might result in a disturbance in the secretion of insulin, and that this in turn might contribute to atherosclerosis and diabetes.

Underlying all this was his assertion that modern diets have diverged from the ancestral norm. In his book *Pure, White and Deadly* he wrote: "It does matter that your diet is now very likely to be different from that which has been evolved over millions of years as the diet most suitable for you as a member of the species *Homo sapiens*" (Yudkin 2012, 5). Initially published in 1972, although it raised the profile of the sugar problem at the time (see e.g. Cleave 1974), the book was unable to topple fat as the dietary public enemy number one. Nevertheless, it was revised and republished in 1986 and again in 2012 following renewed interest in the problems posed by dietary sugar, promoted, among others, by Professor Robert Lustig, the American paediatric endocrinologist at the University of California, who then published his own book on the subject: *Fat Chance: Beating the Odds against Sugar, Processed Food, Obesity, and Disease* (2013).

A study published in 2014 by James J. DiNicolantonio, an associate editor with the *British Medical Journal*, also warned that sugars, especially those added to processed foods and fizzy drinks, pose a greater threat to the heart than added salt, and are more likely to cause high blood pressure, stroke and heart disease (DiNicolantonio and Lucan 2014). Heart disease is the number one cause of premature death in the developed world, accounting for some 350,000 deaths in the United States and costing more than US$50 billion each year. Compelling evidence implicates sugars, especially the monosaccharide fructose, as playing a major role in the development of high blood pressure. One culprit the study cites is high-fructose corn syrup, frequently used as a sweetener in processed foods, particularly fruit flavoured and fizzy drinks. The consumption of such sugar-sweetened beverages has been implicated in 180,000 deaths worldwide per annum. Some 300 years ago, individuals only consumed a few pounds of sugar a year, but current estimates suggest that average consumption in the United States is up to 150 pounds a year. Of particular concern is that teenagers in the UK and the United States may be consuming up to 16 times the recommended limit for added sugars. The research notes that naturally occurring sugars found in fruit and vegetables are not harmful to health; it is just the modern industrially produced products that are.

Meat

Professor T. Colin Campbell found another possible culprit for those 'western diseases', which he identifies in his book *The China Study* (Campbell and Campbell 2005): for him it was the consumption of animal protein, meat and dairy products, that seemed to lie at the root of the problem. His book was named after a major study of the dietary habits of some 6,500 villagers (50% male, 50% female) drawn from 65 rural counties in China. Those results were then compared to the records of mortality rates, incidence of cancer and other diseases from the surrounding regions during 1973–1975. The study included a comparison of the prevalence of western diseases (coronary heart disease, diabetes, leukaemia and cancers of the colon, lung, breast, brain, stomach and liver) in each county. The study collected and collated diet and lifestyle variables (ignoring all other factors) and found that as blood cholesterol levels rose, so did the prevalence of western diseases. The conclusion drawn by Professor Campbell was that long-term health benefits to Chinese and other Asian people who have traditionally existed on a primarily plant-based diet might be lost as more people switched to a western-style diet that was richer in animal-based foods.

But was it the animal-based foods or was it other aspects of western-style urbanisation that were the real culprits? Denise Minger (2013) has forensically charted the protracted battle between these nutritional heavyweights and the controversy over the differing roles played by fats, sugars and meat in the development of the diseases of affluence. She has, for example, comprehensively deconstructed many of the arguments mounted in *The China Study* that seemed to support Campbell's central proposition. By scrutinising the initial data sets, rather than the statistically averaged general statements, she showed that the evidence collected in the study on the rise in the consumption of animal protein did not actually correspond with a rise in disease, even in the highest animal food-eating counties – for example, Tuoli. Indeed, Frank B. Hu and Walter Willett (2002) also re-evaluated the data, and unequivocally state that the survey of 65 counties in rural China did not find a clear association between animal product consumption and risk of heart disease or major cancers.

Minger also points out (2013, 135–137) the key reasons why these detailed studies were unable to provide a crystal clear answer to the question of what is the main dietary factor leading to or predicting cardiovascular problems. And this was because the wrong question was posed: heart disease is more complex than that, and diet is just one issue in a complex system that crucially involves environment, culture, activity regime and individual genetics. Consequently there may not be one simple answer or one simple cause. Fat and cholesterol metabolism differ from person to person, most notably those that carry the ApoE4 gene. Chimpanzees and some other primates also have a version of this gene, and thus it must have been in our genetic make-up for at least six million years. In times of scarcity, this gene would have helped cholesterol from dropping too low by boosting the body's ability to retain as much dietary fat and cholesterol as possible. However, in our modern, more abundant times, those who have this gene with its inherent storage capacity (rather than its variants ApoE2 or ApoE3) have a significantly higher risk of not only heart disease but also Alzheimer's. It's not always what you eat: it can be simply who you are (Minger 2013, 133–135).

The wider academic nutritional controversy rages on, and with it the battle for public health and accurate dietary advice. James J. DiNicolantonio authored and co-authored a number of papers in 2014 with scientists who believe that a diet including saturated fat does no harm to most human hearts. In the same year, Frank Hu led the 2015 Dietary Guidelines Advisory Committee's report on saturated fat and cardiovascular disease (USDA 2015). The guidelines have now changed from recommending low fat to recommending moderate fat.

A diet to live for

Table manners

Modern diets differ dramatically from ancestral norms: the calorific density, glycaemic load and intake of added sugars are all much higher, whereas our micronutrients, dietary bulk, fibre content, long-chain fatty acids and protein intake are all less than what our uncivilised genes assume is normal (Konner and Eaton 2010). Nevertheless, it is often suggested in some quarters that the adoption of a 'Palaeolithic diet' and exercise regime is little more than a fad. There is still a confusion between diets designed to lose a few pounds after seasonal Christmas overeating and regimes that underpin a healthy long-term lifestyle. Western society has also been bombarded with the promotion of 'super-foods' and a series of celebrity-endorsed diets. These include the one proposed by Herman Taller in 1961 which avoided all carbohydrates; the one developed by Robert Atkins in 1972 promoting protein-rich meals over carbohydrates; the South Beach diet which selected particular carbohydrates and fats and avoided others; the Mediterranean diet, advocating fruit, vegetables, olive oil, fish and unrefined grains (see e.g. Simopoulos 1999, 2000); Pierre Dukan's list of some 100 'allowed' foods; while Mark Hyman (Cleveland Clinic Center for Functional Medicine) has promoted the Pegan diet, combining aspects of a Palaeo diet with aspects of veganism. Another celebrity-endorsed diet that could claim to have a direct connection to the evolutionary determinants of health is that based on our blood groups, O, A, B or A/B, a development promoted by Dr Peter D'Adamo.

In spite of inherent contradictions, it has been shown that the aspects of these regimes that do prove effective are working directly or indirectly with the evolutionary determinants of health – our Palaeolithic physiology and metabolism. Take, for example, Michael Mosley's fasting diet, developed in conjunction with Professor Mattson from the American National Institute of Aging. If you have no food for 24 hours – perhaps a not uncommon occurrence in some seasons during our long past – your energy needs will transfer from depleting the supply of glucose in your blood to the energy stored in your liver, and after that, to burning off fat. Such a system is designed to support the body in genuinely lean times: it will work equally as effectively if confronted with a proxy-failed harvest (i.e. a self-induced fast) and consequently could help those suffering from obesity. Table 5.1 evaluates examples of 'fad diets': the Atkins diet (Atkins 2002) promotes a high-protein/low-carbohydrate regime, while the Ornish diet (Ornish 1993) recommends the reverse. The contrasting composition of these two diets is shown. They are compared with a reconstructed 'standardised' hunter-gatherer regime (see O'Keefe and Cordain 2004, table 1) and the 'Mediterranean diet' (e.g. Simopoulos 2000), which is rich in fresh fruit and vegetables, fish, olive oil and unrefined grains.

Table 5.1. Comparison of a hunter-gatherer style diet with a low-carbohydrate, a low-fat and a 'Mediterranean-type' diet

	H-G	Low carb (Atkins)	Low fat (Ornish)	Mediter-ranean
A				
Protein (%)	H: 19–35	M: 18–23	L: <15	M: 16–23
Carbohydrates (%)	M: 22–40	L: 4–26	H: 80	M: 50
B				
Total fat (%)	M: 28–47	H: 51–78	L: <10	M: 30
Saturated fat	M	H	L	L
Monounsaturated fat	H	M	L	H
Polyunsaturated fat	M	M	L	M
C				
Omega-3 fat (fish/ nuts)	H	L	L	H
D				
Total fibre	H	L	H	H
Fruit and veg	H	L	H	H
Nuts and seeds	M	L	L	M
E				
Salt	L	H	L	M
F				
Refined sugars	L	L	L	L
Glycaemic load	L	L	H	L
H-G = Hunter-gatherer; L = Low; M = Moderate; H = High				

Source: O'Keefe and Cordain 2004, table 1.

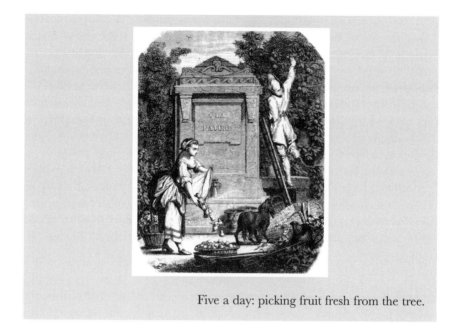

Five a day: picking fruit fresh from the tree.

A different approach

So where does all this controversy and the ambiguous results of all these expensive studies lead us? Unambiguous evidence-based research is demanded by governments and national health authorities if statutory dietary guidelines are to be issued or altered. Acceptable bodies of evidence, correctly interpreted, are usually based on detailed, statistically significant studies, recording various variables such as smoking, incidence of cancer and age at death. The participants (human or animal) would normally form two groups – for example, a smokers group and, to provide a control, a non-smokers group. A longer term longitudinal study would involve a large cohort (or cohorts) whose health has been tracked over time to identify correlations and hopefully potential causes of particular diseases or conditions. A number of such studies have been mentioned in this chapter and the interpretations of the results discussed. But a different approach, working from a different standpoint, will now be introduced.

A robust a priori case can be made for simply accepting that ancestral diets, refined by millennia of natural selection, have proved their worth by supporting humankind for two or three million years or more; a longitudinal study par excellence with a global distribution. The necessary control group is provided by the well-documented rise in western lifestyle diseases found in modern urbanised populations. The research questions posed are to what extent do our modern dietary regimes differ from an evolutionary-concordant datum, and what are the health consequences of such divergence?

The study of the relationship between the ancestral and the modern diet has a long history of its own, as the work of Weston Price (1939) shows. But it was much enlivened by debates that were associated with the period of plenty that followed the Second World War when diets changed profoundly. Not everyone agreed that this was a change for the better: in Austria, for example, Dr Wolfgang Lutz dealt with health issues related to the high-carb diet enjoyed by thousands of his patients. The assessment he published in 1967 suggested that we should turn our backs on the staple product of the Neolithic Revolution and restrict our daily carbohydrate intake to just 72 g: a life without bread (*Leben ohne Brot*) (Allan and Lutz 1967). Work by Hugh Trowell and Denis Burkitt over a 20-year period in the 1950s and 1960s, in clinics in Kenya and Uganda, confirmed the observation that 'western diseases' were not prevalent in the native populations (Burkitt et al. 1974; Trowell and Burkitt 1981) and led to the concept of the high-fibre diet.

An American gastroenterologist, Walter Voegtlin, was also unhappy about his patients' health and, as a result of his work on colitis, Crohn's disease and irritable bowel syndrome, he suggested that a diet based on what he thought ancient hunter-gatherers enjoyed would cure many of the ills he faced in his surgery. His landmark book, *The Stone Age Diet*, was published in 1975, but it seems to have over-emphasised the role of meat. Anthropologists such as Dr Vaughn Bryant (of Texas A&M University) revised the approach (e.g. Bryant 1979, 1995) at a time when further study of Palaeo nutrition was advancing significantly in university departments across the globe (e.g. Wing and Brown 1979; Brothwell and Brothwell 1998).

By 1985, that message had been taken forward on a broader front in an influential article in the *New England Journal of Medicine* by physicians S. Boyd Eaton and Melvin Konner from Emory University (Eaton and Konner 1985). This was followed up by two popular books, *The Palaeolithic Prescription: A Program of Diet and Exercise and a Design for Living* in 1985 and *Stone Age Health Programme* in 1989. Professor Loren Cordain from Colorado State University, now a leading advocate of the Palaeo diet (2012 [2002]), was introduced to the concept after reading Dr Eaton's seminal paper. Since 1984, a prime research focus for Dr Artemis P. Simopoulos has also been on evolutionary aspects of diet. She has written, co-authored and edited many volumes on nutrition and obesity, and has been editor of the influential Karger 'World Review of Nutrition and Dietetics' series since 1989 (see e.g. Simopoulos 1999). Her output also includes popular books on the Omega diet (Simopoulos and Robinson 1998) and a paper on the Mediterranean diet (Simopoulos 2000). This distinguished founder and president of the Center for Genetics, Nutrition and Health in Washington, DC has taken a particular interest in such issues as the essential fatty acids and the omega-6/omega-3 balance, and how modern cultural changes have adversely impacted upon it (Simopoulos 2006).

Perhaps the most comprehensive study inspired by Eaton and Konner's 1985 report was initiated in 1989 by the Swedish doctor Staffan Lindeberg. The Kitava study surveyed the population of an island in Papua New Guinea which had no incidence of stroke, ischemic heart disease, diabetes or obesity (Lindeberg and Lundh 1993). A series of papers have subsequently been published examining the so-called Palaeolithic, ancestral or pre-agricultural diet in comparison with the modern dietary regime and its associated diseases. This influential research culminated in the ground-breaking study *Food and Western Disease: Health and Nutrition from an Evolutionary Perspective*, published in English in 2010. The book is an evidence-based study compiled over 20 years, and it lists no less than 2,034 academic papers in its bibliographic references. The result is a persuasive argument for serious consideration of the damning role played by our western diet in coronary heart disease, stroke, atherosclerosis, type 2 diabetes, obesity, insulin resistance, high blood pressure, dyslipidaemia, heart failure, dementia, cancer, osteoporosis, rickets, iron deficiency and autoimmune diseases.

Thus, over the last 30 to 40 years, the benefits of 'ancestral-style' diets have gained medically authoritative references and a wide academic readership, certainly in the United States. An increasingly large number of books have popularised the concept, sometimes by the researchers themselves (as listed above) and sometimes by others extending the idea – or at least elements of it – to an ever widening audience (e.g. Chaitow 1987; Audette 1995; Sissons 2009; de Vany 2011). It should be stressed that not only has the medical research studying the benefits of such diets increased, but also the archaeo-logical and anthropological evidence that underpins the work continues to clarify and expand our knowledge of the dietary regimes in question (e.g. Ungar 2006; Gremillion 2011; Kiple and Kriemhild 2012; Kelly 2013).

In the 25 years following the publication of the influential *Palaeolithic Prescription*, the authors have developed their thesis and provided counter-arguments to its detractors (Konner and Eaton 2010). Perhaps more importantly, they have also evaluated subsequent research on how departures from the nutrition and activity patterns of our hunter-gatherer ancestors have contributed significantly to the endemic chronic diseases of modern civilisation. They have concluded that ancestral human diets prevalent during our evolution, when compared with today, were characterised by much lower levels of refined carbohydrates and sodium and much higher levels of fibre and protein. Comparable levels of primarily unsaturated fat and cholesterol, however, were balanced by much higher levels of physical activity (Konner and Eaton 2010).

In addition to stressing the crucial link between diet and exercise, they also record that concerns are now being raised about the once common official recommendations that argued for very low levels of protein, fat and choles-terol intake. Thus a series of conventional epidemiological, clinical and laboratory studies conducted over the last quarter of a century have leant solid support to the concept that a proxy-ancestral diet might well prove widely beneficial. Indeed, official recommendations today now have targets moving rather closer to those prevalent among hunter-gatherers than did comparable recommendations 25 years ago (Konner and Eaton 2010, 594–602). The two once separate dietary research trajectories, one medical, one evolutionary, are now happily converging.

Solutions and resolutions

Medical and nutritional scientists have devoted many years to studies that aimed to identify the associations between particular foods and particular diseases and conditions. The ultimate aim was to provide evidence-based research that underpinned unambiguous advice promoting good health through the adoption of healthy nutritional regimes and, of equal importance, identifying foodstuffs associated with poor health outcomes. Major concerns were the often wide divergences of expert opinion: by way of example, Loren Cordain records that in 1996 the American Society for Clinical Nutrition and the American Institute of Nutrition concluded that the intake of trans-fatty acids was *not* a risk factor for coronary heart disease. In 2002, however, the National Academy of Sciences, while debating the increased risk of cardiovascular disease, recommended that trans-fatty acid consumption should be kept as low as possible (see Lindeberg 2010, viii).

To take a more positive line, a selection of studies that support the principal tenets of the ancestral diet, even though they were not necessarily conducted with that concept in view, are summarised below.

Good fat, bad fat

Possible links between poor cardiovascular health and diet have been the focus of many studies. A review of over 100 such reports (Hu and Willett 2002) suggested that, contrary to some accepted dogma and some public health guidance, it was not the intake of meat, cholesterol or total fat that seemed most to blame. Based on the evidence presented, the authors argued that the regimes which provided the most positive support for cardiovascular health were those that avoided a particular fat type, the saturated fats, such as those found in fried foods, most pre-packaged industrially processed snack foods and commercially baked products. They suggested that these should be replaced with fats that have a positive, beneficial impact on our health, such as the monounsaturated and polyunsaturated fats (see Table 5.1) from products as readily available as nuts, a favoured item in many hunter-gatherer diets. Nuts such as almonds, hazelnuts, pecans, pine nuts, pistachios and walnuts contain particularly high levels of the 'good' fats that can lower harmful fats in the blood, and thus can give similar benefits to patients who might otherwise be prescribed cholesterol-lowering drugs or statins. Eating a handful of nuts, an apple or taking four tablespoons of extra virgin olive oil provide an effective alternative to statins for preventing heart attacks for those in the low-risk categories (Malhotra et al. 2015).

It has also been argued that walnuts, if eaten regularly, can improve cognitive functions such as memory, concentration and the speed at which information is processed. An associated study looked at a large US sample population with ages ranging from 1 to 90 years old, part of the National Health and Nutrition Examination Survey (NHANES), which has consequences for those concerned with slowing or even preventing the progression of conditions such as Alzheimer's. There are a number of active ingredients in the walnut that might be contributing to the positive results, since it has a high antioxidant content, contains a range of vitamins and minerals and is the only nut with a plant-based omega-3 fatty acid (Arab and Ang 2015).

Polyunsaturated fats such as omega-3 are naturally present in algae, grass and leaves, and are thus absorbed into the food chain by many creatures on land and sea; humans historically benefitted from omega-3 through the consumption of fish and the lean meat of the larger grazing animals. Regrettably, the fattier meat of modern domesticated creatures that are grain or corn fed is lower in omega-3 than that of their free-ranging cousins in the wild (O'Keefe and Cordain 2004, 102–105).

Of relevance to this issue are recent studies on the significance of the ratio between omega-6 and omega-3 fatty acids in our diets. Anthropological and epidemiological research suggests that human beings living as hunter-gatherers developed a dietary regime with a balanced omega-6/omega-3 ratio of 1:1, whereas in most modern urbanised populations the ratio is between 15:1 and 17:1, with much higher levels of omega-6 in the diet. This is the direct result of two changes: first of all, we are eating far less omega-3 rich foods such as fish, poultry, nuts and grass-fed animals. But we are consuming far more products with high levels of omega-6, such as those containing processed vegetable oils like sunflower oil, corn oil and soybean oil, although olive oil, coconut oil and palm oil are all relatively low in omega-6.

The distorted omega-6/omega-3 ratio in modern dietary regimes is alarming, since it seems to be associated with the development of many chronic conditions. This is a consequence of changes related to how the body processes these two different types of essential fatty acids (EFA). Omega-6 fatty acids have a pro-inflammatory effect on the body, while omega-3 fatty acids are anti-inflammatory. Ingesting rather too much of the former negates the necessary bodily balance, and leaves us open to the development of cardiovascular disease, diabetes, some cancers, autoimmune diseases, rheumatoid arthritis, asthma and depression (Simopoulos 2006). This is another dramatic example of how our ancient physiology, metabolism and digestive systems are unable to accommodate to the drastic changes in dietary regime so suddenly developed by the modern world. It is yet another evolutionary determinant of our health or, if we maintain the abnormal 15:1 to 17:1 ratios, an evolutionary determinant of our ill health.

As a worrying postscript, there are even more problems with cooking oils and fats: when they are heated the chemical composition can change through oxidisation, and potentially dangerous aldehydes and lipid peroxides are produced. These are known promoters of cancer, heart disease and dementia when eaten or even inhaled. A controlled experiment by Professor Martin Grootveld (De Montfort University, Leicester) tested sunflower oil, vegetable oil, corn oil, cold-pressed rapeseed oil, olive oil (refined and extra virgin), butter, goose fat and lard to see which ones were the most and least culpable in this regard (Grootveld et al. 2014). Contrary to initial expectations, he found that oils which were polyunsaturated-rich, such as corn oil and sunflower oil, which are fine when cold, when heated generate very high levels of aldehydes. In contrast, the olive oil and cold-pressed rapeseed oil produced far fewer aldehydes; more surprisingly, so too did butter and goose fat. These are richer in monounsaturated and saturated fats, and are much more stable when heated. It is worth recalling that all the refined vegetable oils are modern inventions: none were available in prehistory. But lard was.

Green party

A recent study suggested that changing to a vegetarian diet might be able to cure diabetes in some cases. This is extraordinary news for the three million people who suffer from this condition across the globe. Diabetes can lead to blindness, amputation, heart disease, kidney failure and stroke and, according to the World Health Organization, is currently set to become the seventh leading cause of death within the next 15 years (WHO 2016). The new study started from the assumption that removing animal fats from the diet improves insulin sensitivity, and therefore focused on the nutritional regimes of vegetarians and vegans. It was suggested that a vegetarian diet can significantly improve blood sugar levels and manage type 2 diabetes, since such diets reduce levels of a blood-protein called glycated haemoglobin (HbA1c). For diabetes sufferers, the higher the HbA1c in their blood, the greater the risk of developing diabetes-related complications. The researchers therefore analysed the dietary patterns of 255 adults with type 2 diabetes who had changed to a low-fat vegan diet or a no-meat diet that included eggs and dairy products. They reported a lowering of HbA1c by an average of 0.4 percentage points and sometimes by as much as 0.7 points (Yokoyama et al. 2014). This is a comparable effect to that produced by prescribing drugs such as alpha-glucosidase inhibitors that help to control blood glucose levels by preventing the digestion of carbohydrate. This was a relatively small-scale experiment, and it cannot be proved that the trigger was not the cessation of meat eating rather than the increased consumption of vegetables. Nevertheless, this study does demonstrate the positive elements of plant eating; disregarding such a key element of an ancestral diet arguably increases the risk of type 2 diabetes.

Medical research has also demonstrated that nitrates help to reduce blood pressure and regulate the body's metabolism. Some recent studies by the Universities of Southampton and Cambridge have shown that a diet including beetroot or green leafy vegetables such as spinach (all rich sources of nitrates) is especially beneficial in this regard, since it can reduce the production of a hormone called erythropoietin. This is made by the liver and kidneys and determines the quantity of red blood cells we have, how thick our blood is and how much oxygen can be carried around the body. Too many red blood cells in the system can lead to thickening of the blood and to hypoxia, a common symptom in many cardiovascular diseases (Ashmore et al. 2014b). Eating more green vegetables can not only help to alleviate those symptoms, but also those of many other heart and circulatory diseases. This is because such a diet also increases the production of compounds that allow the heart to pump more efficiently, by widening our blood vessels (Ashmore et al. 2014a). Further research has shown that nitrates also stimulate the conversion of 'bad' white fat cells into 'good' beige fat cells, a process that can reduce the risk of obesity and type 2 diabetes (Lee et al. 2012). Clearly, ignoring the evolutionary determinants of health and not eating your greens is bad for you.

Seven-a-day

Consuming more, rather than less, vegetable matter has even more to commend it, as the next two examples show. Analysis of the records of 1,200 participants in the Jiangsu longitudinal nutrition study over the period from 2002 to 2007 has thrown light on a particular health concern, that of multi-morbidity. This is an increasingly common condition, especially in the elderly, in which the patients suffer from two or more chronic medical problems simultaneously. The challenge for the medical profession is that treatments for one problem often exacerbate the other(s). The study, by a team based at the University of Adelaide, looked at links between diet and 11 chronic diseases including anaemia, hypertension, hypercholesterolemia, diabetes, arthritis, hepatitis, coronary heart disease, asthma, stroke and cancer. Data were adjusted to take into account differences in age, sex, BMI, marital status, sedentary lifestyle, smoking status, annual income, education and energy intake. The authors concluded that "greater consumption of fruits and vegetable and whole grain products appear to lower the risk of multimorbidity" (Reul et al. 2013). Another recent study, this time by the University of Queensland, suggests that eating eight or more portions every day also dramatically improves mental wellbeing. Dr Redzo Mujcic collected data from 12,000 Australian adults to examine how their consumption of fruit and vegetables correlated with their mental health. It would seem that women experience a greater mental health benefit than men, and that fruit has a larger impact than vegetables on mental health (Mujcic 2014).

Thus, the benefits of eating plenty of fresh fruit and vegetables and avoiding foods with quickly digestible carbohydrates and a high glycaemic load is now widely accepted and appears in most health authority dietary guidelines. But how reliable are those guidelines? Way back in 1990, the World Health Organization published its recommendations for healthy living, suggesting that we should be consuming 400 g of fruit and vegetables every day (WHO 1990). In 2003, the UK government launched its own initiative, the now famous 'five-a-day' advice, in common with France and Germany. Australia, however, suggested a more generous '2 and 5' items that incorporated two (150 g) portions of fruit in addition to five (75 g) portions of vegetables. This grand total of 675 g is significantly larger than the UK recommendation.

Major research conducted at UCL by Dr Oyebode and her team seems to suggest that the Australian approach – consuming rather more vegetables and fruit – should be followed (Oyebode et al. 2014). The study examined the records of some 65,226 individuals recorded in the Health Surveys for England over the period 2001–2008. All the participants were aged 35 or over, forming a statistically significant random sample of the non-institutionalised population, the health of which was tracked over a seven-year period. A relationship was sought between the consumption of fruit and vegetables and mortality, whether by cancer, cardiovascular disease or other causes of death, but adjusted for age, sex, social class, education, BMI, alcohol consumption and physical activity.

Eating not five but at least seven portions of fresh fruit and vegetables a day was linked to a 42% lower risk of death from all causes, a 31% lower risk of heart disease or stroke and a 25% lower risk of cancer. It was the fresh vegetables that seemed to provide greater protection against disease with each daily portion reducing the overall risk of death by 16%, a portion of salad by 13% and each portion of fruit by 4%. Our physiology has been adapted to collect, eat and digest a daily complement of fresh vegetables and fruit; the evidence-based research discussed here provides proof that our digestive systems have not, as yet, evolved beyond that of the hunter-gatherer. Taking this standpoint, Dr Oyebode's research shows not only that eating more vegetables increases your chance of a longer life, but also, more worryingly, that the more your diet diverges from a Palaeolithic norm, the shorter your life is likely to be.

In terms of modifying modern national health behaviours to better fit our biology, these findings strongly support the Australian approach to your daily fruit and veg ration (2 and 5). This may be compared to the less generous UK advice (just five a day) which also recommends that frozen and tinned fruit may be included in the daily allowance. Alarmingly, the UCL study suggests that these particular sources may be better avoided, since those who regularly ate canned or frozen fruit actually had a higher risk of heart disease, stroke and cancer. It should be stressed, however, that the survey data available to the researchers unfortunately did not differentiate between frozen and tinned fruit. The current assumption is that the adverse health effect was probably not related to the frozen foods but to the additional sugars and syrups added to the canned products, although more research must be done to clarify this.

Sweet tooth

This brings us on to our love affair with sugar. This too has its roots in our hunter-gatherer past, for when a fruit was ripe enough to eat it would taste sweet to the Palaeolithic palate. However, sundry cooks, confectioners and food manufacturers have subsequently benefitted from this evolutionary signal. By adding sugar to their dishes, they fool us into thinking that their food is as nutritious as fresh fruit, when in reality it makes us obese (and them a profit). Only by conscientiously avoiding such unnecessary additives, and selecting foodstuffs more in keeping with the metabolism we have inherited, will our bodies remain healthy and fit for purpose. At one time, the battle for healthy living focused on lowering the fat content of highly processed foodstuffs, and many low-fat products appeared on the market. However, many of these had extra sugar added to them to sharpen the flavour and bulk them out. A current bone of contention is now concerned with the detrimental role played not just by fats, but by sugar (sucrose/fructose/dextrose) in the health of modern urban populations. Most authorities agree that too much is indeed bad for you, but government advisers, the food industry and independent researchers are unable to agree on the amounts that can be consumed without compromising an individual's health.

A World Health Organization report in 2015 looked at the health impact of sugar, including damage to teeth, the increasing prevalence of type 2 diabetes and the effect on obesity. In a marked change to the position it held in 2002, the World Health Organization now recommends that the proportion of sugar in our diet should be below 10% of our total calorie intake (50 g per day for an adult of normal weight), while stressing that a figure of 5% should be the target. These limits apply not just to sugars naturally present in honey, syrups, fruit juices and fruit concentrates, but to those subsequently added to all foods and drinks. Public Health England's director of nutrition and diet, Alison Tedstone, claimed that their own surveys show that the UK population should reduce their sugar consumption very dramatically, as the average intake for adults is 11.6% and for children is 15.2%, well above the current UK recommendation of 10% (Tedstone 2016). Some, such as the campaign group Action for Sugar, are pressing for 5% to become the firm recommendation. Should there be more clearly defined limits to the amount of sugars added to industrially prepared foods (perhaps with more aggressive labelling)? Should adding sugar solely to bulk up foodstuffs cheaply be banned outright? Even Dame Sally Davies, England's chief medical officer, has hinted that highly sweetened products might have to be taxed at a level that could dissuade consumers from purchasing them in ever larger quantities (see Borland 2014). What is clear is that our bodies were simply not designed to accommodate such abnormally high levels of sugar, any more than they can cope with decades of inhaling noxious cigarettes.

Resorting to the law

Organisations such as the proactive Public Health England have a concern with, and a responsibility for, 'improving' our health and addressing the urban lifestyle diseases that blight so many lives. Challenges to our Palaeolithic physiology, such as smoking, irresponsible drinking and eating foods with too high a salt and sugar content, have to be attacked on several fronts: the producers, the advertisers, the shops and the consumers. It's not just about blanket bans, but about the provision of suitable substitutes in a culture that believes in individual freedom and the value of a free market economy. The battles to stop drink-driving and to ban smoking in public places have been very long drawn-out affairs, with influential vested interests unwilling to act for the public good unless or until the law demanded it. In Europe, for example, there is the Common Agricultural Policy (CAP): all European member countries are obliged to conform to this framework of food pricing and production processes. It has been noted that the burden of diet-related disease has grown considerably since it was first implemented; the policy concerns market measures and rural development rather than the relationship of food to its citizens' long-term health (NICE 2010, recommendation no. 8). Negotiations to change the focus of the CAP to take a more evolutionary-compliant stance to food and diet are unlikely to be straightforward.

Meanwhile, the war on foods and drinks with added sugar continues (see e.g. Lustig 2013; Minger 2013). The damage to teeth is terrible. In 2013–2014, for example, some 26,000 UK children aged between 5 and 9 were hospitalised for multiple tooth extractions, a figure which had increased from previous years, according to the Health and Social Care Information Centre

(HSCIC 2015). Should we be replacing all our children's teeth with sucrose-resistant dentures, or just removing the sucrose? But it's not solely a dental challenge, as sugar added to drinks and food products is clearly still in the frame with regards to the war against obesity, diabetes and cardiovascular disease.

The now obsolete Carbohydrates Working Group, part of the UK government's Scientific Advisory Committee on Nutrition (SACN), finally recommended in 2015 that our sugar intake be limited to 5% of our energy intake, a figure which mirrors that already proposed by the World Health Organization. However, the scale of this challenge is highlighted by the UK's national diet and nutrition survey, as this shows that 15% of the calories consumed by 4- to 10-year-olds comes from sugar, while for 11- to 18-year-olds the figure rises to almost 16%, with fizzy drinks and fruit juices the main sources (DoH 2012). Advertising such products to children may have to be stopped and a 20% tax on products with added sugar may be required to curb consumption. France has already imposed such a levy on soft drinks, and the UK is set to do the same following statements made in the budget in March 2016, targeting drinks with over 5 g of sugar per 100 ml at one level and those with more than 8 g of sugar per 100 ml at an even higher level.

Producers need to reformulate their ingredients and stop adding extra sugar to soft drinks (perhaps incrementally over time, as was done with pre-salted foods): Michelle Obama has championed such a drive in the United States, where companies such as Kellogg's, Nestlé and Pepsi have been working to cut 6.4 trillion calories from their products over a five-year period. Coca-Cola and the makers of Cadbury's chocolate are also reformulating products (although they are not saying by how much), as are some British companies, such as Britvic and Tesco, and this has seen the removal of some ten billion calories in a year. This proves what is possible from the food manufacturer's standpoint. As for the UK's producers of sugar beet, their situation also needs to be addressed if their industry is to be modified: perhaps they should change their focus and consider the market for biofuels or switch to growing fruit and vegetables.

Needless to say, the World Sugar Research Organisation (which is funded by the sugar producers themselves) will continue to fight such measures, even contesting the evidence-based research underpinning proposals from the World Health Organization (which is not funded by the sugar producers). Nevertheless, one of the prime evolutionary determinants of health is that our bodies don't need added sugars and most certainly cannot cope with them. The archaeological and anthropological evidence is clear; the results of the rationing of sugar during the Second World War are clear; the evidence linking sugar intake to obesity levels is clear. But, in spite of many behind-the-scenes initiatives and media campaigns for and against, it may well take further legislation to get sugar off the shelves.

All things are possible: if we were to adopt an evolutionary-concordant nutritional regime designed to suit our own individual genome, then we would not have to reject all the benefits and opportunities that tomorrow's urban living may offer. We can remake modernity: our behaviours can be re-normalised, our townscapes reconfigured and even our foodstuffs reformulated. We can, literally, have our cake and eat it (provided it has an evolutionary-concordant recipe).

Chapter 6

BODY OF EVIDENCE

Lack of activity destroys the good condition of every human, while movement and methodical physical exercise save it and preserve it.

Plato (*c.*428–*c.*348 BC)

Irregular exercise

It has been said that the sofa has contributed to the death of more people than the motor car. A study in *The Lancet* published in July 2012 suggests that the alarming increase in physical inactivity, particularly in modern cities, has had a major health effect worldwide. The following statistics make sobering reading for those of a sedentary disposition: "physical inactivity causes 6% of the burden of disease from coronary heart disease, 7% of type 2 diabetes, 10% of breast cancer, and 10% of colon cancer" (Lee et al. 2012). The report concludes that of the 57 million deaths that occurred worldwide in 2008, the deaths of more than 5.3 million people could have been averted just by regular exercise.

But rather than demanding furniture manufacturers stand trial for crimes against humanity, a searching look at our modern urban culture and our basic biology is required. Activity regimes, like nutrition, are key evolutionary determinants of our health. This simple message needs constant promotion: walking to work (as with more strenuous sports) is as good for the mind as for the all-too-often sedentary body of today's city dweller. Public Health England, along with the Department of Health and the National Institute for Health and Care Excellence (NICE), have also expressed major concerns at the developing obesity epidemic. This is a chronic disease that leads to premature death, and is directly linked to an increased risk of hypertension, colorectal cancer and type 2 diabetes, by five times in men and by twelve times in women. A survey published in 2014 showed that two-thirds of English adults were overweight or obese (i.e. they had a BMI of 25–30 or more), as were one-fifth of all children aged just 4 to 5 years old (DoH 2014).

Sedentary modern urban lifestyles are very different from the daily activity levels that our Palaeolithic genome anticipates (see box 'Working out', page 94). The sixth of the eight-point guidance on healthy living provided by the National Health Service is simply "Get active and try to be a healthy weight". In a speech made in Sheffield in January 2013, Baroness Susan Campbell, the head of UK Sport and the Youth Sport Trust, was alarmed by the statistic that 20% of children starting primary school are overweight and by what she has termed the "physical illiteracy" of children starting secondary school, still unable to throw or catch a ball, run or jump. She argued that such a situation does not bode well for the nurturing of future sports stars, and it also does not bode well for the National Health Service. Our primary schools clearly need to take a more evolutionary-compliant approach to education; that means training not just the modern mind, but also the ancient body.

Working out

A study by Professor James H. O'Keefe and his research team from the University of Missouri explored elements of the hunter-gatherer activity regimen that should be considered by anyone wishing to develop guidelines for an evolutionary-concordant modern urban lifestyle (O'Keefe et al. 2011): some of the key issues are summarised here. The report included observations from anthropologists such as Professor Kim Hill (Arizona State University), who lived and worked with the Aché hunter-gatherers of Paraguay and the Hiwi foragers in Venezuela.

- The human race is genetically adapted for a life of routine activity rather than for long sedentary periods. Walking, lifting, bending, climbing and carrying (wood, water, food and children) all proved essential for survival.

- The actual tasks that needed to be accomplished in a 'normal' hunter-gatherer's day would vary depending on factors such as the level of hunger, the season, the weather or the terrain. Nevertheless, a typical distance covered by human locomotion might be in the range of three to ten miles per day. The necessary daily activities would require (on average) an energy expenditure of between 3,000 and 5,000 kJ, perhaps as much as five times greater than many modern sedentary adults (Cordain et al. 1998).

- Given the physical demands of their daily life, hunter-gatherers were usually lean and rarely obese: this reduced trauma to joints and minimised diet-induced inflammation. But a body designed for a life of walking, as well as bending, lifting and carrying heavy loads, needs to undertake such activities regularly; if the skeleton is not so used, then osteoporosis, osteopenia or sarcopenia might ensue.

- In the past, most walking and running would have been done barefoot and on grass or mud. Such activity contrasts with urban jogging on concrete in expensive, restrictive running shoes. Some recent studies are beginning to question the overall health benefits of such modern artificial exercise, given problems such as shortening and stiffening of the tendons and foot ligaments, plantar fasciitis, ankle sprain, Achilles tendonitis, hamstring tears and lower back pain (Bramble and Lieberman 2004; Lieberman et al. 2009).

- In addition, these vigorous activities would have been done primarily in the open air, rather than in the confines of an air-conditioned gym, as is often the case today. Outdoor exercise helps to maintain ultraviolet-stimulated vitamin D production in the epidermis which, among other benefits, can improve mood.

- Social interaction and cohesion were part and parcel of the daily round for hunter-gatherers: regular tasks associated with hunting and gathering were usually undertaken as group activities.

- Music, rhythm and dancing were (indeed are) key components in virtually all tribal societies, forming the basis of active communal celebrations and ceremonies.

- A particularly strenuous day for hunter-gatherers could be followed by a relatively easy one or a storm event might prohibit too much activity. Days of rest, imposed or not, were important, helping the body to recuperate in readiness for future endeavours.

- Dogs/wolves have been co-evolving with humans for very much longer than creatures such as sheep, cattle or horses. Semi-feral wolves may have helped in the hunt for several millennia before being used to round up flocks and herds. Walking the dog, a common contemporary urban activity, is thus not only beneficial for our health, but has a deep ancestry.

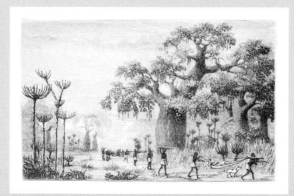

For hunter-gatherer communities, the daily demands of obtaining sufficient food, firewood, water and so forth necessitates mobile, active lives.

Lifestyle-embedded physical activity

Medical research repeatedly shows that many health problems can be directly linked to diminishing activity levels in an urban culture that is so different from that for which our bodies evolved. A research project conducted in North America tried to address the question of how much less active modern populations are than they were in the past. The angle taken was a novel one. The activity levels of four groups of 8- to 13-year-old children were compared: one group was from a school in urban Saskatchewan and another from a rural community in the same state. The results from these contemporary groups were then set against children who were often leaner, stronger and with less evidence of obesity than the Saskatchewan schools. One of these groups was from an Old Order Mennonite school, a community which enjoyed a lifestyle that had changed little over the last 60 years. The fourth group came from an Old Order Amish school, a farming community which embraces simplicity and 'traditional' values, where the ownership of cars, bicycles, tractors and telephones is still not permitted. In other words, they represented a lifestyle that was commonplace some 100 years ago. The study showed that modern lifestyles seem to be associated with pronounced lower levels of moderate and vigorous intensity physical activity. Although this shortfall could be made up with additional sports and so forth, it was noted that the prime difference seems to be the physical nature of lives dependent on farming and on many manual chores. It was these lifestyle-embedded physical activities, rather than jogging, gyms or organised sport, that provided the levels of exercise required for a 'healthy life' (Esliger 2010).

Active evolution

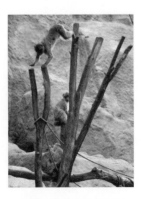

Figure 6.1. Branching out: these macaques, like most Miocene apes (our ancestors), spend much of their time foraging in the trees.

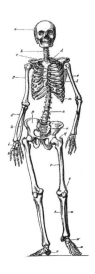

Figure 6.2. Stepping out: note the length and strength of human leg bones, which are designed for walking.

But active lifestyles were not just the product of hard-working 19th-century lives. According to crucial DNA evidence and further archaeological studies, a clearer picture is emerging of how and when our anatomy developed the way it did. We now know that our gene stock can be traced back over seven million years to an ancestral line shared with other primates. Many of these earliest primates spent much of their lives climbing trees: swinging from branches was the standard mode of propulsion in the constant search for food and security. It is now thought that the last common ancestor of humans and chimpanzees still moved on four legs when on the ground. However, some four million years ago our human ancestors were walking upright, as fossilised footprints in Tanzania prove. This was a profound evolutionary development or mutation, showing that we were now ground-loving creatures. The gradual physiological evolution of this new posture saw the skull balanced on the top of the spine, which developed a slight curve, while the hips became broader, the legs longer, the feet now had arches and the big toe became aligned with the rest of the foot (unlike the thumb and the hand). There is also a gap between the top of the pelvis and the bottom of the ribcage: this is not occupied by a large gut (the sort associated with a bulky plant-based diet) since this area was required for the abdominal muscles needed to keep the frame upright. These new creatures therefore needed a rich high-protein diet, such as one containing meat. In other words, walking upright (bipedalism) required a major anatomical reconfiguration in terms of the skeleton, the muscle attachments and the posture.

It is one of the defining characteristics of the human frame (rather than that of all our ape-like relations) and cannot represent a sudden overnight change. In other words, modern humans are very clearly designed physiologically to walk, as opposed to swing through branches or sit in cars all day. Since that part of our design seems to have remained largely unchanged for some three to four million years, we can deduce that walking or running were essential attributes of the ancestral daily round. Human locomotion was thus the principal means whereby the territory from which all essential food and resources must be won would have to be traversed each and every day.

However, recent research has identified some unwelcome skeletal differences between hunter-gatherers and more modern humans. In a study by Timothy Ryan (Pennsylvania State University) and Colin Shaw (University of Cambridge), skeletal remains representing individuals from four distinct human populations, ranging from mobile foragers (hunter-gatherers) to more sedentary agriculturalists, were compared with each other and with some 30 extant primates. It seems that bone strength in the hip joints of the mobile hunter-gatherers was comparable to non-human primates of a similar size, but was significantly more robust than the agriculturalists (Ryan and Shaw 2014). These results show how particular aspects of our bone structure can be directly related to differing activity levels and therefore, by extension, how a more sedentary lifestyle reduces bone strength and increases the risk of fractures.

Further research by a team led by Professor Christopher Ruff (Johns Hopkins University, Baltimore) took that conclusion forward, and considered when and why our mobility levels decreased to such a level that it impacted on our bone strength relative to our body size – that is, our skeletal robusticity. The remains of 1,842 individuals from northern Europe dating from the Upper Palaeolithic (some 11,000 to 33,000 years ago) to the 20th century were examined, and the relative strength of the upper and lower limb bones calculated and plotted across time. This work identified when the most significant decline in the bending strength of the tibia and femur in the legs first occurred, after which the human skeleton gradually took on the more gracile features with which we are now familiar. The most marked change was between about 4,000 and 7,000 years ago. This was the period we now call the Neolithic, when more sedentary patterns of agricultural life were first adopted. Communities were now able to harvest their daily food requirements from a smaller territorial area, and so, in addition to marked dietary changes, mobility levels also began declining (Ruff et al. 2015).

Not only were plants domesticated but so too were animals: cattle and sheep could now be corralled rather than hunted, another saving in human energy expenditure. Just as significant was the taming and breeding of horses and other creatures to become beasts of burden. This lightened the loads our ancestors had to carry and enabled them to travel greater distances faster and with relatively less effort.

The Neolithic Revolution underpinned major changes in territoriality and socio-political organisation, while the rise of urbanisation saw the division of types of labour along gender and class lines, as well as a greater susceptibility to infectious diseases. Many fundamental aspects of the hunter-gatherer culture were supplanted as these key cultural and agricultural changes took hold and spread ever further. Such was the universal impact of these revolutions that they even changed our anatomy: our skeletal robusticity would never be the same again.

Give me sunshine

Vitamin D is another evolutionary determinant of our health. It is essential for the body, since it enhances our ability to absorb calcium, iron, magnesium, phosphate and zinc. Unfortunately, few foods contain vitamin D, and thus exposure of the skin to sunlight is the normal way to obtain this crucial benefit for us, as for most mammals. This is an important factor, and not just for those considering exercise in a gym rather than in the great outdoors. In modern cities where families live in apartments with no outside space, or where children are not allowed to play outside for fear of crime or cancer, and where the dietary regime is poor, vitamin D deficiency can and will occur. This is a serious condition, and can take the form of osteomalacia or rickets in children. In addition, a study of over 7,000 British adults showed that the levels of vitamin D were alarmingly low during the winter and spring, a situation that needs to be addressed at a national, rather than an individual, level. Perhaps even more worrying is that, in western urbanised populations, pregnant women are identified as a high-risk group. The consequences of severe clinical vitamin D deficiency in these women can be life threatening to the newborn, and can also have important long-term health implications for the surviving offspring (Hyppönen and Power 2007). Regardless of how urban we have become, our uncivilised genes still expect us to live active lives in the great outdoors.

Exercising the brain

Sedentary behaviours are not just bad for the body but bad for the brain, since they deprive it of improved neuroplasticity and neurogenesis: exercise helps the brain to grow. A comparative study was made of the muscular strength, cardiovascular fitness and IQ of 1.2 million youths entering military service in Sweden from 1950 to 1976. The scoring ranked them at the ages of 15 years old and then 18 years old, and subsequently tracked them into adulthood. Interestingly, the data set included 270,000 brothers and 1,300 identical twins. The study showed that the better predictor of cognitive ability and IQ was not, as might be expected, the familial relationship, but their cardiovascular fitness (Ratey and Manning 2014, 109–110).

Exercise not only promotes mental agility but also mental health, as James Blumenthal's seminal experiment at Duke University showed in 1999. His study concerned three groups of patients being treated for anxiety or depression. Group one were given anti-depressants, group two began a regular exercise regime and group three tried both. After ten months, those in group two who were still exercising were clearly better off than those in group one just taking the tablets (Blumenthal et al. 1999).

To sleep, perchance to dream

Active days are one thing, but we all still need sleep to recuperate, to allow the body to repair and rebuild itself. And the brain also demands adequate downtime to process the information it has absorbed during the preceding day. In antiquity, this was all part of the natural cycle, the circadian rhythm of night and day, before such differences were dissolved by electric lights and the working demands of 24/7 cities. We know that there are two basic levels of sleep, the first accompanied by rapid eye movement (REM), the second, the deeper stages of non-REM sleep. The following summary of research related to the evolutionary determinants of sleep is taken largely from John Ratey and Richard Manning's illuminating chapter in their book *Go Wild* (2014, 125–150). They describe how hunter-gatherers used to sleep in the open, in the wild, but communally, in groups or families. To offer protection from many nocturnal predators, someone had to be awake or needed to be a light sleeper. As it happens, different age groups have different sleep patterns which are shared in cultures across the globe. Adults differ from adolescents (who go to bed later and sleep longer) and from older people who are often awake for longer during the night, and also from babies with their random wake-up-at-all-hours cycle. Thus in a 'normal' mixed tribal community of, say, 35 people, someone will naturally be on sentry duty without the need for a formal rota. Sleeping communally made sense and helped keep you safe (and thus facilitated your deepest, most productive sleep), until at least part of that guard duty could be performed by dogs. Modern epidemiology has shown that people who are married or who have pets live longer than those who live on their own: is it the companionship that makes the difference, or is it the improved quality of the shared sleeping (Ratey and Manning 2014, 140–145)?

Detailed sleep-deprivation studies were made by the US military as a consequence of campaigns forcing soldiers to work outside standard nine-to-five hours. The loss of sleep led to craving very dense carbohydrates and sugars, such as the ubiquitous Snickers bar. These results have been confirmed in the civilian world, where sleep-deprived students gained weight by eating more as the body's 'normal' recuperative sleep cycles were disrupted. There are also, unfortunately, impacts on our ability to perform even simple tasks, to recall facts and to solve problems. Individuals with a good night's sleep ultimately prove their worth over self-styled, over-caffeinated over-achievers operating ineffectively on four hours' sleep a night (Ratey and Manning 2014, 128–131).

But there is an even worse problem looming for the sleep deprived, as a recall study all too graphically demonstrated. Emotionally charged positive, negative and neutral images were shown to two groups, one sleep deprived and one not. When later asked to recall those images, the first group had significant difficulty recalling all but the negative images, a situation clearly linked to depression. Another study, equally illuminating, was of clinically depressed people who also suffered from sleep apnoea (a breathing difficulty that prevents sleeping). Once medication had successfully treated the breathing problem, the ensuing natural, normal sleep promptly cured the depression (Ratey and Manning 2014, 131). All these studies prove that another evolutionary determinant of your active wellbeing is, somewhat ironically, eight hours' sleep a night.

Chapter 7

A LIFE LESS SEDENTARY

The journey of a thousand miles starts with a single step.

Mao Zedong (1893–1976)

Active life

Although it's exhausting just to think about it, our energetic ancient ances-tors probably expended between 3,000 and 5,000 kJ on a normal day. Such a figure is not often exceeded by many modern urbanites (Cordain et al. 1998), and certainly not in the average trip to the supermarket. It is this low level of activity as much as poor dietary choices that leads to poor long-term health. Inventions such as the TV, the car and the personal computer have all contributed to the seemingly unstoppable rise in obesity levels among urban populations. None of these factors are directly responsible: it is the culture surrounding them and how we use, or overuse, them that is the issue. Taking the discussion of all these elements one stage further, how easy is it to develop an activity regime that is evolutionary concordant but can be readily incorporated into a sedentary urban lifestyle?

It seems there are at least three approaches to the challenge. The first one would establish daily/weekly exercise programmes based on how many kilojoules of energy need to be expended, how many miles need to be walked or run, and how many hours of sustained aerobic exercise and resis-tive training should be completed to attain the required levels of fitness. In other words, how to bolt an artificial activity on to your daily routine that would counterbalance and correct the negative effects of the sedentary life currently being enjoyed.

The second approach would be to modify that sedentary lifestyle itself by incorporating and embedding far more physical activities into your everyday life. Walking all or part of the way to work or school, for example, would make human locomotion a normal and necessary part of your daily round, rather than just something to be measured on a treadmill.

The third way would be a compromise of the first two: try to incorporate/add as much activity as possible into your everyday life (e.g. don't take the lift), but be keenly aware of where the gaps are so that artificial exercise can be resorted to in order to top up when required. And, of course, it should not be forgotten that activity and nutrition are intimately linked: the types and quantities of food consumed will directly determine how much energy could be at your disposal. You are what you do and you do what you eat.

Whatever the exercise regime you choose, it has to be regular. Daily walking is ideal, or cycling or swimming, together with lifting, stretching, bending and running upstairs; a variety of everyday exercises can be enjoyed (or endured) without joining a gym. Contrary to popular opinion, sustained jogging, marathons or gym-based power training are less beneficial for the long-term health of most ordinary mortals, since such intense levels of activity cannot be sensibly sustained, and therefore should be left to the training of professional athletes. At heart, the discussion revolves around how pragmatic (or how clinical) you are, and whether you wish to evolve a 21st-century lifestyle that builds directly upon your basic biology or whether you feel that you can supplement your modern life with additional activities, just as you can supplement your diet with vitamin pills. To take an extreme example: if you wish to expend 837 kJ, you could run for 15 minutes on a treadmill or you could spend half an hour in vigorous sexual activity, pushing your heart rate up to over 120 beats per minute, and maybe seeing your systolic blood pressure rise up to 200 mm Hg (O'Keefe et al. 2011, 477–478). Both are evolutionary-concordant ways of 'keeping fit': one is arguably artificial, the other is arguably normal, but both will work.

On benefits

Sustrans is a UK charity that promotes sustainable transport options such as cycling and walking. Its leaflet 'Why Walk? Step Your Way to a Happy, Healthy Lifestyle' (2009) lists the benefits of walking, including:

- For adults, 30 minutes of walking five days a week dramatically cuts the risk of developing heart disease, diabetes and some cancers.

- Walking reduces cholesterol, lowers high blood pressure and raises your sense of wellbeing.

- Walking burns as many calories as jogging over the same distance.

- Unlike running, walking is a low-impact exercise that does not stress the knees.

- Walking is free.

- Walking rather than driving is good for the environment, since not using the car reduces CO_2 emissions and urban air pollution while making streets quieter and safer.

Promoting cost benefits in London

Cost benefits could become a major factor in the promotion of active commuting (i.e. walking to work or school). Londoners use smartcards (called Oyster cards) to pay for underground and bus journeys. These cards are pre-charged, and there are differential rates for daily, weekly or monthly seasons, which also vary in price according to the number, more or less, of the concentric zones through which the commuter passes. The charges are currently weighted in such a way that the more you travel on public transport each day, the cheaper each journey becomes. There is therefore no direct cost incentive to walk even part of the daily commute. Would a solution be to offer a reduced price for a weekly or monthly season for those who actually travel less on the bus/tube and walk more?

Daily exercise or daily grind?

The terms 'regular exercise' and 'lifestyle-embedded activity' need to be distinguished from the actions that cause repetitive strain injuries. In our ancient past, daily life involved a wide variety of different actions, rather than the repetition of a single action over and over again. The latter routines became ever more common after the adoption of large-scale agricultural practices and the subsequent development of towns: such settlements had an increased dependence on the specialisation of crafts and trades, and the associated if often mind-numbingly repetitive activities required. There are sound evolutionary reasons why our attention span is thought to range from a few seconds to 20 minutes or so: any creature living in the wild cannot afford to be so involved with a task that they are oblivious to the potential dangers that could be stalking them. We haven't lost that essential psychological defence mechanism, and neither has our anatomy adapted to such unnatural activity patterns: repetitive strain injuries involving the arm, shoulder and neck affect some 30% of workers in modern urban societies. Approximately one-third of all compensation paid out to workers in the United States was for such injuries, for example (RSI Therapy 2005). The condition can be associated with many tasks involving the repetition of forceful exertions, mechanical compression or sustained working in awkward positions, such as prolonged work at a keyboard set at the wrong height. And even the fittest athletes can suffer from golfer's elbow (medial epicondylitis) or tennis elbow (lateral epicondylitis) and other conditions resulting from over-repetitive demands on the musculoskeletal and nervous systems.

Your regular activity regime, like your diet, should be varied and should not be monotonous; it should exercise and strengthen your anatomy, rather than deform it (see e.g. Bowman 2015). Why we need to exercise our Palaeolithic bodies daily is now clear. Regular physical activity in the fresh air in a green or greened environment is an essential component of a normal evolutionary-concordant lifestyle. Clearly we are not exercising enough, but how can the behaviour of a whole urban population be changed for the better? Is this just a personal choice, does it require a deeper cultural change, and what can the state do to promote greater levels of physical activity? Then, to take matters to another level, how might buildings and even town plans be reconfigured to better fit our biology? These are some of the issues discussed and debated in this chapter.

Human locomotion

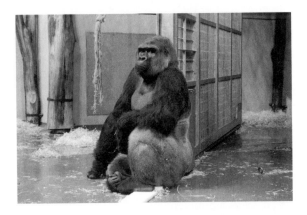

Figure 7.1. Life in the slow lane? The human frame was not designed for long periods of inactivity.

As part of the continuing programme to promote increased activity levels, a series of guidelines have been published by Public Health England (NICE 2008a, 2008b, 2009, 2010, 2012). These reports also detail how regimes involving lifestyle-embedded activities such as walking and cycling might be better built into the urban environment (e.g. PHE and LGA 2013; TfL 2014). This requires more than rewriting Sir Ebenezer Howard's treatise on garden cities (Howard 1902), which was compiled in an age before the automobile ruled, for settlements today are very different animals, in scale, function and population density. It is not just poor dietary choices that can lead to poor long-term health, since most of us also need to lead less sedentary lives. What is clear is that the design of our public transport systems, our buildings, our streets and our townscapes can significantly help us to achieve that goal, and get us back to the levels of daily exercise that our

Palaeolithic physiology expects. Walking or cycling to and from school, or at least for part of the daily route to work and back, would be a simple solution to reducing weight and health problems while also providing significant psychological uplift (Martin et al. 2014). If such a programme was universally adopted on a city-wide basis it would also reduce car travel, traffic congestion, air pollution, carbon dioxide and diesel emissions, noise levels and road traffic accidents.

Changing behaviour: reinventing the foot

On the face of it, the official guidance seems straightforward enough: if you are relatively active on a daily basis and walk at least a mile or two (that's less than an hour) each day, you will live longer, be more healthy and be less of a burden on the National Health Service and on society in general. But, of course, life is never that simple. A study called 'Understanding Walking and Cycling' was undertaken from 2008 to 2011 to look at the factors that influenced everyday travel decisions for short trips in urban areas – that is, the very trips for which walking (or cycling) would seem most suited. By compiling a list of the negative issues raised, the research team thought it would be possible to suggest the ways and means to address or overcome them, and then to implement the appropriate policies on the ground (Poole 2012).

The detailed survey was conducted in the four English cities of Lancaster, Leeds, Leicester and Worcester, and 1,417 responses were returned and analysed, supported by a number of interviews. The aim was to probe the reasons why people who claimed they would like to undertake more active travel failed to do so. Three specific themes seemed to be most common. The first related to concerns about the physical environment, with potential cyclists in particular being worried about heavy traffic. The second was shared by many with young children, and was the perceived difficulty of slotting walking or cycling into complex household routines, juggling commitments with the moving of (tired) children, the paraphernalia needed for such journeys and parental concerns about safety. For many, taking the car seemed the simpler, easier option. The third reason is perhaps the most interesting, and might well underpin both the first two rationalisations. This is that, for many, walking and cycling are in some way abnormal things to do in a culture where car use is habitual, normal and convenient. In other words, if all your neighbours drive the kids to school, why should you stand out as the only ones who walk?

Once again the chicken and the egg have arrived: it seems clear that if more people walked or cycled, then even more people would walk or cycle. Indeed, this does seem to be the case in areas where human locomotion is increasingly seen as normal, therefore others will certainly follow. So how can you square the circle? Colin Poole's report makes seven recommendations that address the challenge of facilitating behaviour change. Several of these concern town planning issues such as establishing safe, designated cycle tracks, making pedestrian route-ways welcoming and restricting traffic speeds to 20 mph in residential areas. Another comments on the need to develop more neighbourhood shopping centres (rather than the out-of-town superstore versions that demand cars), and the provision of secure bicycle parking facilities in town centres and bike storage units in most homes. Then there was discussion of the introduction of wider societal and economic changes that would give people the flexibility to undertake more active travel, with family-friendly working hours and so forth.

But the final recommendation concerned the third major theme raised in the survey itself: the necessity of changing the image of walking and cycling through campaigns to promote active travel as normal, acceptable and accessible to all (i.e. not just for the keep-fit fanatics). That concept, the rein-vention of the foot, requires cultural change, not just behaviour change, although the other facilitating measures summarised above could be part of the solution.

Poole's study suggested there should be concerted campaigns to get more people walking. In fact, there have been several (see e.g. NICE 2006); some were aimed specifically at getting kids to walk to school (or rather aimed at persuading parents to stop taking their offspring in the car) (NICE 2009). Certainly, a more effective way of promoting active lifestyles is to embed the concept of walking as a normal activity in children from the outset. The charity Living Streets have taken up the challenge of persuading children, parents and teachers that walking is good. Figures from the social trends section of the Office for National Statistics for 2009 and 2010 note that only 50% of primary schoolchildren walked to school in 2009, down from 62% in 1991, and thus that trend needs arresting and reversing. According to the Living Streets website, their Walk to School initiative has reached 13 million people, and thus is seen as one of the UK's largest behaviour change pro-jects for young people. The team already work with 750,000 children and with 2,000 schools, while many thousands more took part in other events, such as the national Walk to School week in 2013.

These projects also address particular safety problems that are thought to hinder the extension of the scheme. Indeed, the majority of walking chil-dren aged between 7 and 10 are accompanied by their parents, who cite fear of assault or molestation and traffic danger as particular concerns. Living Streets have therefore campaigned about issues such as pavement parking (where cars are driven onto the often narrow pavements, forcing children and parents with buggies into the road), increasing the time limits of pedes-trian crossings, arguing for funding for the lollipop people (the team who loyally man crossings outside schools) and pushing for 20 mph speed limits on residential roads, especially those around schools. All these issues, if resolved, would help to remove obstacles that adults feel make walking to school unsafe for children. Staying with the parents, it is also clear that their familiarity with the neighbourhood and its occupants could also be a positive or negative factor in whether or not a child would be allowed to walk to school, regardless of well-kept gardens, trees or traffic-calming measures.

And then there is the concern over distance: in London, with its tightly drawn catchment areas, the majority of children live within a reasonable walking distance of a state school, but this is not always the case elsewhere. A study in North America, for example, highlighted the problem of the closure of many older, smaller 'neighbourhood' schools over the last 40 years: now only one in five live within 1.6 km of their school (Gilliland et al. 2012). To promote the school walk here would require more than just the greening of streets, but the planning and construction of accessible schools and their immediate locale to encourage safe and sensible human locomotion.

Changing streets

To further encourage such major cultural changes as persuading an urban population to actively commute to work, solid modifications to the townscape are required. People prefer to walk in city centres with wider pavements, pedestrianised routes and well-designed shared spaces, or through parks, quieter or greened back streets, with good street lighting and CCTV at night time. Roads that pass through shopping centres should have traffic calming measures or a 20 mph speed limit. Many cities are now implementing designated cycle networks (with the attendant cycle racks, signage and major road crossing points), and work has begun on extending that principle to pedestrians. In Wales, Cardiff is developing its Walkable Neighbourhood Plan (www.keepingcardiffmoving.co.uk), identifying a network of streets and parks that serve key local destinations to positively encourage walkers, part of a wider programme developed as part of the Active Travel (Wales) Act 2013 (see Welsh Government 2016). The associated guidelines appeared in the same year that Lucy Saunders and her team published their highly impressive Transport Action Plan for London (TfL 2014).

Proof that cars and their fumes are a real deterrent for pedestrians is shown by projects such as the Ciclovía, initiated in Bogotá, Colombia, but now increasingly common in many cities elsewhere. On Sundays, many main streets are simply closed to vehicular traffic and given over to human locomotion, an altogether pleasanter urban experience. From this it follows that wide pavements combined with traffic calming (or exclusion) can be powerful architectural statements in the drive to get people back on their feet. One of the ultimate pedestrianisation schemes was the 5 km long Promenade

Plantée in Paris, which saw transformation of the disused elevated Vincennes railway line into a tree-lined parkway, with arts and crafts shops occupying the arches of the former viaduct below for part of its course. It was completed in 1993, and was the inspiration for several other similar urban schemes, such as the Atlanta BeltLine (Georgia, USA), a 33-mile multi-use path along a disused railway that now connects 45 neighbourhoods with 1,300 acres of public greenspace. Perhaps the most famous example is the High Line in New York: work on the obsolete Central Railroad began in 2006 and continued in stages until 2014, running (or walking) from West 14th Street to 30th Street.

In the UK, planning authorities now have responsibilities that move beyond the regulatory role in controlling land use activities to that of a "place-enabler and place-shaper" (PHE and LGA 2013, 2). Street-shaping requires thought, interaction with the communities involved, planning and resources. Some of the funding can (and does) come from the developers of major urban sites, through what are known as Section 106 agreements (that being the number of the relevant section in the Town and Country Planning Act 1990). Planning permission for a redevelopment may only be granted if a condition of that permission is the obligation to provide a cycle path, greenspace or other public amenity that can be factored into the wider urban network.

Then there is the relatively new Community Infrastructure Levy (CIL). This is a tax on development, the purpose of which is to fund infrastructure, and is based on a fixed charging schedule that relates to the size of the building project. The use and impact of this levy is as yet unproven, but presumably it could be utilised to help make key routes more attractive for pedestrians. The Equality Act 2010 requires public authorities to make reasonable adjustments to improve access for those with more limited access, sight or hearing. This can involve the removal of cluttered street furniture (e.g. guard rails, bins, bollards, wheelie bins in inappropriate places) as well as the redesign of, and better placement of, pedestrian crossings. The Localism Act 2011 introduced new rights for communities of residents and local businesses to work together through a neighbourhood forum or parish council to suggest improvements. Last but not least is the Public Services (Social Value) Act 2012, which obliges public bodies to consider how, for example, the carrying out of works would improve the economic, social and environmental wellbeing of the community involved. Taken together, there is therefore an effective legislative and planning framework to support moves to improve our streetscapes on evolutionary-concordant lines, making streets greener and more welcoming for social interaction and for active travel. If communities wish to change their neighbourhoods for the better, then they are now allowed to do so.

Back to the gym? by Matt Morley, founder of Biofit

Any attempt at defining an evolutionary-concordant approach to fitness is coloured by the fact that 'physical fitness' as we think of it today is an inherently modern concept. For much of the past 2.5 million years being fit for the task of survival was all that mattered. The daily movement required for hunting, gathering, fishing and self-protection, interspersed with well-earned rest periods, wasn't an optional lifestyle choice, but was at the heart of life itself. Seen in this light, the concepts of calculated reps and sets, of exercise and participating in sports as pastimes, need to be recognised for what they are: luxuries bestowed upon us by civilisation. An evolutionary-concordant interpretation of fitness, on the other hand, requires the avoidance of routine – variety of movement is key. Evolution also rewards practice: once you've worked out how to hit a moving target with a rock or defend yourself from attack, there's only one way to get better at it. Play is evolution's in-built mechanism to encourage practice during downtime, play-fighting being a way for children to develop familiarity with necessary robust life skills, for example.

Rather than limiting ourselves to specific workout times, we'd do better to look for ways to integrate regular, low intensity movement into our daily lives, such as walking, cycling, gardening or playing with pets. This serves as a baseline. Many such activities will likely take place outside, providing an additional opportunity to reconnect with nature, nourishing the soul and calming the mind in the process. Going barefoot enhances this effect further, waking up the feet in response to the undulations and textures of the land beneath.

Whereas most fitness today is focused on form over function, muscle over movement, by working with a variety of locomotions, not just walking but crawling and suspending patterns, we force the body into what are now unfamiliar positions. Similarly, functional strength is best developed via compound, multi-joint movements with a clear purpose, such as pushing oneself up from the ground, pulling oneself up on top of something and lifting a heavy object using either a squat or hinge motion, then carrying it and placing it in a new position.

The 'fight or flight' concept also takes us in two additional directions. Fighting skill is an oft-neglected element in primal fitness, but the ability to protect oneself and one's tribe from attack played a larger role in our ancestors' survival than many care to admit. This may sit uncomfortably for some today, but the armies of martial arts fans around the world are tapping in to that in-built warrior mentality each time they step onto the dojo mat. The lighter side of fighting is, as already mentioned, play – a largely undervalued adult activity that helps us to develop new neurological pathways, reaction times and hand–eye coordination. As it is often dependent on a willing partner, it also offers myriad opportunities for interaction, light physical contact and fun.

However, flight has more day-to-day relevance for most of us. A degree of cardiovascular capacity, along with strength and mobility, are the building blocks upon which all real-world fitness is built. A realistic flight situation would equate to a short sprint at one extreme, to be practised several times with short rest intervals, while a distance run intended to cover more ground would be at the other. Both have merits and both have their place in a complete evolutionary-concordant training regime.

Finally, seeking out ways to move, lift, sprint, crawl, climb and play/fight within the considerable constraints of modern western lifestyles presents real challenges. Consequently, relearning how to move as nature intended demands a concerted effort to reset the accumulated tightness in our wrists, shoulders, hips and ankles that results from too little activity and too much sitting in adult life. Arguably, a regime incorporating outside activities as well as dedicated gym space may be required. It's not a quick process, of course, but from an evolutionary perspective at least, we have plenty of time to fix it.

Changing buildings

Designing a town that encourages and facilitates physical human locomotion and other physical activities is not just about external spaces, streetscapes and the public realm, it's also about the internal design of the workplace. There is now clear evidence that a sedentary office life, involving many hours of sitting down, is linked to increased health risks. A pioneering study of the comparative health of 31,000 sedentary bus drivers and active bus conductors published over 60 years ago made this point tellingly (Morris et al. 1953a, 1953b). Both groups of employees worked for the same company and came from the same social class. The study showed that the drivers not only had a higher incidence of coronary heart disease, but even more worryingly, they were twice as likely to die as a consequence than the conductors.

There have been many other subsequent studies of such sedentary drivers, all underlining the dangers. A study from the Netherlands showed that bus drivers were four times more likely to develop disablement from musculoskeletal disorders when compared to civil servants (Kompier et al. 1990), while a study from Sweden showed that bus and taxi drivers had the highest ratio of coronary heart disease when compared with 30 other occupations in a group of nearly 7,000 males (Rosengren et al. 1991). The situation was no better in Taiwan, where an investigation of over 2,000 males showed that the drivers had higher rates of obesity, hypercholesterolemia, hypertriglycer-idemia and incipient heart disease than a control group of skilled workers (Wang and Lin 2001). Reading such a catalogue as this, it is clear that the workers whose jobs demand that they are seated for prolonged periods every day suffer a very high risk of coronary heart disease.

But being a driver is not the only job that requires sedentary postures for long periods. A recent publication has reported on the effects of sitting occu-pations on the health of over 10,000 men and women drawn from English and Scottish health survey cohorts (Stamatakis et al. 2013). The participants were classified as standing, walking or sitting during their work time, and the results were monitored against a range of attributes including age, general health, levels of drinking and smoking, social class and educational back-ground. In the 12-year period in which the study was conducted, 754 deaths were reported. Statistical analysis of the results showed that, compared to those in standing or walking occupations, there was a higher risk of mortal-ity from all causes and from cancer for women in sitting occupations.

Other increasingly common approaches utilised in active building design include measures to promote the stairs rather than the lift and introducing standing desks, although those who adopt such a posture must not remain static but remember to keep exercising at regular intervals. Setting up com-munal printing facilities rather than having individual printers right next to the personal computer (thus obliging the worker to walk every time a docu-ment is printed) and having communal staffrooms/water coolers/toilet facilities on different floors also keeps the office moving. The design of the building itself can be made more 'activity-conducive' with the introduction of a 'low-fat' office. Does the building have, for example, sufficient cycle racks, showers and lockers so as to encourage active travel? And it's not just the architecture and layout: the work patterns can also be redesigned (or at least tweaked) to ensure staff are encouraged, or even obliged, to become 'sufficiently active' during the working day.

A similar approach can be taken with the design of schools, in the size and format of classrooms, the relationship of the indoor to the outdoor space, the length of lessons, facilities for physical activities and the amount of time per day that the pupils spend being 'sufficiently active'. It has been shown, for example, that classroom design on its own can have a very significant impact on the learning rates of primary school pupils, based on a study of 751 children working in 34 different classrooms in seven different UK schools (Barrett et al. 2013).

A walk in the park

To develop a physically active evolutionary-concordant urban lifestyle requires personal and cultural changes, all of which come with their own challenges. But, in tandem with that, it would also benefit greatly from hard architectural change: human locomotion should be placed at the heart of town planning policy and reflected in the design of pavements, designated cycle routes, a greater connectivity of streets, an integrated public transport policy and so forth. Residential, public and office buildings should be designed (or redesigned) to meet these needs, as should hospitals and, of course, schools. If the urban environment is especially conducive to active living, then positive cultural change should be easier to promote and progress.

While the benefits of physical activity on our general health are now better understood, there is a growing body of evidence which suggests that being active also has a positive effect on mental health. A long-term study at UCL followed 11,000 people all born in 1958, and recorded their levels of activity in relation to depressive symptoms at the ages of 23, 33, 42 and 50. The research, which was led by Dr Snehal Pinto Pereira from the UCL Institute of Child Health, suggests that those who exercised at least three times weekly were less likely to suffer from depression: the risk was lowered by 16%. Furthermore, it seems that the more they exercised, the more the risk was reduced (Pinto Pereira et al. 2014).

In sum, leading a normal, active life is certainly good for you, physically and mentally (Biddle and Ekkekakis 2005). But the real health message to get across is a negative one: leading an *inactive* life can be fatal. Our modern urban bodies still need a daily workout similar in intensity to that of an uncivilised hunter-gatherer. An influential study compiled for Transport for London calculated that if Londoners chose *not* to adopt an evolutionary-concordant regime of a bare minimum of just 150 minutes of physical activity per week, then such abnormal behaviour could lead to 4,104 more premature deaths, 1,528 extra cases of coronary heart disease, 778 more cases of breast cancer, 474 more cases of colorectal cancer and 44,620 more cases of type 2 diabetes (TfL 2014, 75). It's not just the dog that needs to be taken for a walk each day, every day: it's the human as well.

Chapter 8
LOST TRIBES

He is a barbarian, and thinks that the customs of his tribe and island
are the laws of nature.

George Bernard Shaw (1856–1950)

Social creatures

Having reviewed our uncivilised bodies – what we should eat and what we
should do to normalise our modern nutritional and activity regimes – it's
time for a new challenge. It's not just the physiological elements of our
distant past that remain resolutely Palaeolithic, there's also our mindset,
with the many psychological and societal issues that also impact upon our
present lives. In this chapter, consideration is given to the innate, instinctive
and emotional social responses we still carry with us from our Palaeolithic
past. It is easy to see how aspects of the nurturing of family may have
changed little over millennia – how could it be otherwise? But we have also
retained much of the outlook and many of the imperatives and responses of
the hunter-gatherer, albeit sublimated, redirected or reconfigured for urban
living. The ancient hunter-gatherer's tribal organisation, social structure and
daily survival strategy still underpins much of our urban lives, as hunter-
gathering evolves into a modern world of football and shopping.

But first it's time to consider our uncivilised social brain. Humans are social
creatures, long accustomed to tribal life. Indeed, many other creatures share
such a mentality: flocks of birds, schools of whales, herds of wildebeest and
packs of wolves, for example. Indeed, it has been suggested that the roots for
such sociality can be traced back to the very beginnings of life. In *Global
Brain* (2000), palaeopsychologist Professor Howard Bloom argues that 3.5
billion years ago, bacteria, the early ancestors of all living things, could form
groups of seven trillion or more, while the fossil remains of 500-million-
year-old trilobites are often discovered in mass groupings. There is
presumably safety in numbers.

Our social relations and interactions are as much underpinned by evolutionary needs as is our health. The social units that our ancestors lived and
worked within were family groups or households (parents, children, grandparents), working groups (hunting or foraging parties) and the larger
grouping, the tribe. All would be directly related to a territory from which

their food, water and other resources would be won. That said, there could be movement between groups and between tribes, while the boundaries of territories were established by custom, convenience or enforcement.

Follow my leader

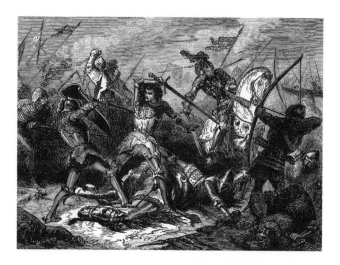

Figure 8.1. Born leader: once such characters were essential in a life-and-death struggle; in peace time the need still survives but is often subsumed in the modern age with, for example, an obsession with celebrities.

As William Wordsworth (1770–1850) observed in his ode 'Intimations of Immortality', children learn much by the process of copying what they see and hear, as if their "whole vocation were endless imitation". The complex process of tribal survival through foraging and hunting in what was often an unwelcoming environment could not be mastered at a stroke: every day, every new situation provided new lessons to be learned. The importance of watching others, and learning by their mistakes as well as their successes, was as crucial for adults as for children. There is therefore within us a need for teachers, for role models, for leaders, at least until such time as the pupils feel ready to strike out on their own. In spite of our new abilities to read, to reason and to access information on every subject under the sun, we have not lost that need: in a modern urban situation it takes on many forms. The cult of celebrity, of film stars, sports stars and pop stars, is more or less a harmless reworking of that drive, bringing with it badges of allegiance and the endless imitation of fashions, hairstyles and codes of conduct.

There is also peer group pressure, the pressing need to conform to current tribal practice. This is more than the exercise of the sincerest form of flattery, for there is strength in numbers. Standing out from the crowd is not always a good thing, since stragglers tend to be vulnerable to predators. The drive is as strong with children in a primary school as it is with fashion- or gadget-conscious adolescents, or with house-owning, car-owning or family-owning middle classes, or yacht-owning upper classes. If you have a tribe, you have to be seen to be part of that tribe, so as the herd moves on, you can't afford to be left behind. Keeping up with the Jones's is part of our innate survival strategy. But if you can't keep up in a large modern city, you can always change tribes.

Then there is the role of the leader, the father or mother figure whose word is law: by dint of hard experience and an innate desire to protect their offspring they know what's best for you, at least in theory. In the household or tribal context, the purpose and function is clear. It is remarkable that in a far more socially complex city or a nation state, we still need a single decision-maker at the top of the tribal tree, however many committees and councils sit between them and their people. It could be a constitutional monarch, a fixed-term president, a democratically elected official, a leader by popular assent or a shadowy power broker, but there always has to be somebody, a person, to head up the tribe: that's an evolutionary determinant. How accountable the 'leader' is or becomes is a political determinant. In a complex society, a hierarchical management structure can, in theory, provide a clear and effective chain of command that can get things done, but should it be the default mechanism for urban society in general?

Band of brothers

Hunting was a key component of ancient communities for the first few million years or so of human evolution, and we still retain the necessary physiological and psychological attributes and drives that underpin such activities. Such hunting parties, normally (but not always necessarily) male, were prepared to pit themselves against unpredictable creatures using cunning and strength in numbers to counterbalance the advantages their adversary might possess. This regular and demanding practice requires patience, knowledge, strength, agility and fast decision-making, not to forget teamwork. It could be a high-risk, high-energy, high-adrenalin exercise: with experience, the risks could be minimised, not just in terms of personal danger, but also in terms of ensuring the success of the expedition for the community's resources.

The more a population visibly expanded, the more boundaries and resources were contested. The inner frustrations of the repressed hunters could then be used to develop warrior bands. This process has been observed in the

Yanomamo of South America, for example, a people who increasingly relied on plantain cropping rather than hunting. The menfolk then developed a graded culture of aggression towards their neighbours, as a result of which periods of peace and amicable relationships could and did degenerate into outright hostility. A natural talent for tracking and killing animals was then used against their fellow humans to settle old scores or steal women (Chagnon 1997, 185–206).

It is also easy to see how, with the gradual development of animal husbandry and sedentary farming, and the associated increased production of non-animal foodstuffs, the need for hunting (as a basic survival strategy) would diminish. There seems little point in arranging long, arduous hunting expeditions if you already have large flocks or herds corralled next to your village. But when men were no longer required to go hunting, the drive and disposition to do so did not simply evaporate. Clearly, those hunters would make ideal warriors should any unwelcome human intruders be found on their territory. Indeed, as ancient society developed and communities expanded into towns, those one-time hunters turned their attentions from wild animals to unwelcome neighbours, and became warriors. In tandem with the need to protect ever growing cities and then to protect or extend enlarging states, these warriors became standing armies.

Urbanisation, slaves and soldiers

Large permanent settlements like cities seem the very antithesis of the hunter-gatherer's world. The archaeological evidence for the origins of urbanisation dates to the Neolithic era, the period associated with the development of farming and animal husbandry (the so-called Agricultural Revolution), which marked the demise of the more ancient and more mobile foraging regimes. As noted in Chapter 3, this process developed independently on various continents at differing dates: now, by utilising these new far more intensive cropping and herding practices, a far larger population can be fed from the foodstuffs harvested from a relatively smaller area. However, the fixed fields that the new agrarian methods demanded had to be defined and defended, as did the domesticated flocks and herds upon which the new communities relied. Land was no longer an open landscape, it became an object to be owned, and those who owned it were unwilling to share, for their lives quite simply depended upon it. The most economical use of the land invited the growth of nucleated settlements, since as the population grew, so more space was required for food production, rather than for sprawling farmsteads and villages.

And so, unwittingly, the foundations were laid some 10,000 years ago for the urban dynamic, the long drawn-out process that saw one sector of society involved in intensive food production, producing a surplus to support other sectors who now had no need to work the land. Those who did not grow their own food contributed to the community through other forms of work as craftsmen or traders, for example.

Slavery: the domestication of humans

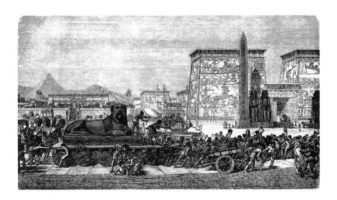

Figure 8.2. Domestication of humans: the history of civilisation is all too often the tale of captured people put to work as slaves or poorly paid labourers.

Way back in 1950, Professor Gordon Childe considered a range of some ten attributes that such early towns might possess, including the development of specialist professions and crafts that only a large centralised population could support or need:

1. Size and density of the population should be above normal.

2. Differentiation of the population. Not all residents grow their own food, leading to specialists.

3. Payment of taxes to a deity or king.

4. Monumental public buildings.

5. Those not producing their own food are supported by the king.

6. Record keeping and practical science.

7. A system of writing.

8. Development of symbolic art.

9. Trade and import of raw materials.

10. Specialist craftsmen from outside the kin-group.

There are at least two elements missing from that list: one is the warrior class, the other the slave class. It is worth recalling that some of the major social changes that the late Neolithic urban revolution brought in its wake still resonate today. The development of the first large social conglomerations that became cities and then empires required the domestication of animals and crops to produce the agricultural surpluses demanded by the expanding populations. And those expanding populations became increasingly socially stratified: the larger the city or empire, the greater the stratification, leading inevitably to a distinct upper class and an equally distinct underclass. This latter development mirrors the Neolithic fate of cattle and sheep, for example, once free creatures whose daily lives and destinies were suddenly under the total control of those who put them to work. This process at the bottom end of the development of social stratification can be described as the 'domestication of humans', the establishment of a disempowered slave or labouring class, the course of whose lives were dictated by the needs of others. And this was not just the harsh phenomenon of Africans being shipped to the Americas to work on sugar or cotton plantations; its shameful history is far older.

The world's first cities or 'civilisations' could not have functioned without slaves: both imperial Rome and even democratic Athens relied on slaves to keep their wheels turning. Even in medieval England from the time of William the Conqueror in 1066, the feudal system saw the crown, its barons, bishops and knights owning all the land, upon which the disempowered domesticated peasantry laboured, beholden to their liege lord for their lives and livelihood. But by a strange twist of fate, it was the late medieval town that offered a route out of this inhumane system. For those who did not work the land but had a trade or craft, could, notionally at least, partially sidestep the central tenets of the feudal system. This might be achieved by working for themselves and their families, as their hunter-gatherer forebears had done before, but now as craftsmen or traders. Thus, although ancient urbanisation may have been the catalyst for extreme social stratification, it could also offer the chance of rewilding, or undomestication, at least for some.

From hunter to warrior

Another feature which was not mentioned in Professor Childe's list of the distinguishing features of early towns was the central role of the warrior. A growing population must not only protect its land from the depredations of its neighbours, but it will also need to enlarge its territory in tandem with its growth. In order to survive and expand, these new urbanised communities needed warriors, without which the boundaries could be breached, its settlements sacked, its valuable livestock stolen and its populations killed or enslaved. It was the hunters-turned-warriors who not only defended the territory but could also extend the boundaries as needs must. This was the calling answered by men for whom hunting was no longer a daily need. For some, warriors are heroes; for most they seemed little more than thugs and the agents of anarchy.

So much of human history has been blighted by the blood shed by these non-hunting hunters. But where would we be without them? The expansion of the great urbanised civilisations of antiquity all required warriors and then armies to underpin them. Such warrior bands were brought together to form the armies of Egypt, Babylonia, Persia, Greece, India, Rome, Carthage and China. All those great civilisations depended on their military might for their success, as much as on their agricultural resources, in a belligerent world with fluid frontiers. The art, culture, political systems and prosperity they created were all predicated on a robust army of men responding to deeply embedded needs to hunt and to follow their tribal leader: the evolutionary determinants of empire.

Born killers? Hunters, warriors and armies

No ancient civilisation could grow without an army to win its wars: none flourished but in the wake of their military prowess, in an age when hand-to-hand fighting demanded ruthless, fearless, well-drilled killers. Thus the very development of every empire owed much to the human hunting psyche. The basic working concept of the Palaeolithic hunting party – the small, tightly knit band of brothers – survived as the core and the catalyst for the urban revolution. It still forms the basic building block in the infantry units of the most modern armies.

For the Roman army, that fundamental unit was the *conturbenium*, a band of eight men who would share not just the same hardships of forced marches and massed battles, but also the same food and the same tent or barrack-block room. Ten of these bands formed a century, six of these a cohort and ten of these a legion. The British army in the recent past also employed eight-man sections, each led by a corporal. Three sections comprised a platoon led by a lieutenant and his sergeant, three platoons a company under a captain and so forth.

Similar systems have been used by many other states in recent times, and seem to represent an almost universal but effective means of command and coordination for infantry armies. Although some communist states have experimented with systems that abolished such rankings (e.g. Soviet Red Army (1918–1935), Chinese People's Liberation Army

(1965–1988), Albanian People's Army (1966–1991)), significantly all felt obliged to re-establish the older, incremental hierarchies to improve operational performance.

This demonstrates that the basic hunting party, led by known individuals, survives subconsciously as a powerful psychological and social force. It was an effective entity one million years ago, and can still be effective today. Thus it can be shown that in spite of major technological advances and breathtaking developments in the scale of operations in two world wars, the foundations of most modern infantry armies rely on the deeply embedded psychology of ancient hunting groups to achieve their aims.

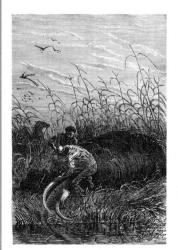
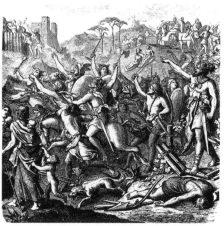
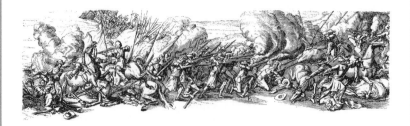

The same mindset that enabled Palaeolithic hunters to track and kill animals for food (top left) was later used by tribal warriors in inter-tribal conflicts over land and resources (top right). Such warrior bands were transformed into larger armies which were able to fight larger and larger wars (bottom).

Polytribal town

It is not just that the structure of an effective modern infantry army works best when based on the core construct of the Palaeolithic hunting party. A contemporary town will also function more cohesively if its social structure mirrors the principles of ancient tribal societies, suitably reconfigured for the 21st century. After all, that is what we are used to emotionally. The population of a great conurbation still think in smaller, tribal-sized units: it is highly significant that some of the most popular TV soap operas recount the lives of modern-day 'tribes', but ones that now live in a particular street, square, village or institution. It's still easier for the human brain to identify strongly with 'tribes' of such an enclosed size: it's a natural reaction. Too large a cast of characters and the engagement fails. This same process is evident throughout our urban lives, for good or ill: in class sizes at school, battling through the rush hour, whether we work in a small family firm or an impersonal call centre; even the number of friends our tribal brains can accommodate seems restricted to about 150 (Dunbar 2014).

A cohesive urban society should therefore not be seen initially as a single entity but more of a collection of sub-units, bound together through an incremental process. Just as our large modern army is a structured conglomeration of small 'hunting parties', so a modern town is best seen as a structured conglomeration of 'tribes' which taken together form a series of sometimes overlapping entities. How this process developed can be seen more clearly in an earlier version of London, as it was between the 12th and 16th centuries. During that period, its population increased to a figure of nearly 200,000, a vast total representing the largest town in the land and one of the largest in Europe. How cohesive was it, and how was that huge urban population structured, mentally and administratively?

The answer to those last questions is that it was subdivided into units, which we will call 'tribes', since that is socially and psychologically what they were. The major cultural development that had taken place since the Palaeolithic period was that Londoners could now happily identify themselves with several tribes at once, since urbanisation required them to take a pluralist approach to tribalisation, to multitask or at least 'multi-tribe': they adapted to the expanding town by becoming polytribal.

Medieval Londoners were polytribal – that is, they were members of many tribes simultaneously. First and foremost, there was the parish: the City had some 111 parish churches at the end of the 16th century. Every Londoner paid tithes to their local church, in return for which the parish priest would marry, baptise and bury them, as well as celebrate mass for them each week. The boundaries of these very pronounced tribal territories were clearly demarcated: everybody knew to which parish each belonged, not least because the tribal boundaries, or parish bounds, were beaten in a communal annual ritual (Wheatley 1956, 434–438; Brooke and Keir 1975, 123–148). Each parish was a distinct neighbourhood in its own right, the City therefore comprising a series of contiguous 'villages', initially organic, self-defining units. These were, in all but name, a medieval version of a Palaeolithic tribe. In this more pious age, the church building itself would form a conspicuous landscape feature in the architecture of the town, its size and embellishment indirectly reflecting the aspirations of the population that supported it.

Parochial City

The earliest churches in the central core of the City (often with smaller parish boundaries) were probably founded in the late 10th or 11th century.

Source: Keene and Harding 1985, pp. xvi–xix; http://www.british-history. ac.uk/london-record-soc/vol22/xvi-xix.

Like all ancient towns, medieval London was a polytribal settlement. It was not perceived socially as just one large tribe, but a series of quite separate communities with which each citizen personally identified. The various tribes every Londoner simulataneoulsy belonged to included their social class (defined by wealth and by dress code in this hierarchical society), their occupation and where they lived. One of the principal tribal determinants was the parish: the City was divided into over 100 such well-defined communities focused on the local neighbourhood church. Medieval London was therefore a series of contiguous tribal 'villages', as shown on the plan above. Such a basic tribal subdivision of a large settlement made it psychologically more comprehensible and thus administratively more workable. The first parishes were built around social units of just 100 to 150 families, a figure that resonated well with the uncivilised hunter-gatherer mindset.

The second City tribe with which each citizen identified was the ward, one of 25 administrative districts, again clearly specified geographically. Membership of this tribe brought military obligations during unrest and also concerned civic matters, both judicial and administrative (Brooke and Keir 1975, 151–153, 162–170). Each ward usually comprised more than one parish, and thus reflected in general terms the administrative unit known as a 'hundred' in the shires or counties outside London.

Both those tribes – the parish and the ward – came with a physical territory, and therefore can be discussed as topographical tribes. By contrast, the next two to be discussed came with a mental or virtual territory. The first of these tribes related to your occupation, perhaps through a craft or trade guild, of which London had at least 80. Many Londoners joined a company or family firm as an apprentice and worked through the ranks for the rest of their life. In some ways it could be argued that the guilds appropriated something of the role or function of the 'lord of the manor' – albeit in an unlanded form – with their large halls, liveries, courts and retainers. Although craft and trade members often lived and worked in close proximity (as the street names of Ironmonger Lane, Bread Street and Vintry imply), there were no long-term fixed boundaries formally set in the townscape for these professional groups. That said, each of these tribes occupied clear conceptual territorial space, with strong, supportive fraternal bonds of membership.

The tribes that constituted the fourth group to be considered were also cultural rather than topographical in terms of the territory they inhabited. These were the tribes that made up the City's social class: London most certainly had a pronounced hierarchy, mirrored by its grand houses, its more modest messuages and its tenanted tenements. The dress and the material culture adopted, as well as the language used (be it French, Latin or Anglo-Saxon), all served to identify each individual's social class – or at least the one to which they were presumed to belong.

In considering these varied tribal units, the location of your house in a particular parish or ward was fixed and finite, and thus so were some of those specific tribal territories. However, some movement was possible (either positive or negative) within your 'virtual' tribes – that is, your class or chosen occupation. As a consequence, neighbourhoods could contain a diverse population of members from differing tribes in the same street. This distinct but fluid tribalisation of the citizenry broke down the impersonal population into social units of a size with which the human mind could more readily engage. This facilitated greater social cohesion, or at least was a system that was conducive to it. As for the communication between these groups, each of the tribes had its 'chief' or spokesperson, be it the parish priest, the alderman, the company master, the lord mayor or the king. Anthropologically speaking, the late medieval town therefore comprised of a series of contiguous parish tribes, each in their own territory or neighbourhood, upon which were superimposed membership of at least three other non-mutually exclusive tribes. The Palaeolithic roots of the complex polytribal urban society were thus clearly in evidence in the medieval City.

City and guilds

Another principal tribal determinant in medieval and Tudor London was your occupation, be it as a labourer, servant, waterman, priest, and so forth. To better regulate the trades and crafts in the City, guilds or livery companies were formed, often headed by a warden overseeing the master craftsmen and apprentices. In 1515, the order of precedence of the top 48 tribes – or worshipful companies – was established thus: mercers (general merchants), grocers (spice merchants), drapers (wool and cloth merchants), fishmongers, goldsmiths (bullion dealers), skinners (fur traders), merchant taylors (tailors), haberdashers (clothiers in e.g. silk and velvet), salters (traders of salts and chemicals), ironmongers, vintners (wine merchants), clothworkers, dyers, brewers, leathersellers, pewterers (pewter and metal manufacturers), barbers (including surgeons and dentists), cutlers (knife, sword and utensil makers), bakers, wax chandlers (wax candle makers), tallow chandlers (tallow candle makers), armourers and brasiers (armour makers and brass workers), girdlers (belt and girdle makers), butchers, saddlers, carpenters, cordwainers (fine leather workers and shoemakers), painter-stainers, curriers (leather dressers and tanners), masons (stonemasons), plumbers, innholders (tavern keepers), founders (metal casters and melters), poulters (poulterers), cooks, coopers (barrel and cask makers), tylers and bricklayers, bowyers (long-bow makers), fletchers (arrow makers), blacksmiths, joiners and ceilers (wood craftsmen), weavers, woolmen, scriveners (court scribes), fruiterers, plaisterers (plasterers), stationers (publishers) and broderers (embroiderers).

Chapter 9

HUNTER-GATHERER VS. FOOTBALL-SHOPPER

Any society does not consist of individuals but expresses the sum of relationships [and] conditions that the individual actor is forming.

Karl Marx (1818–1883)

Polytribalism in the 21st century

So how far removed psychologically from Palaeolithic society is today's urbanised, overpopulated world? And what have football and shopping got to do with our ancestral past? The previous chapter plotted the social trajectory taken (or adopted) by the human race from its hunter-gatherer tribal roots, through the imposition of class and differing work patterns as town life developed in antiquity. It is now time to consider the implications of that study for our 21st-century urban lives. Modern manifestations of the hunting and gathering psyche will be identified, some more socially acceptable than others. But first the bigger picture will be painted. It is argued here that a modern town, whatever its size, needs a similar polytribal social structure to that described for medieval London if it is to function as a cohesive, inclusive entity. How such a framework is scaled up from a settlement of 50,000 to one of five to ten million while still integrating the key elements is the real question.

Although specific location can be important, such multi-layered, pluralistic, tribally based systems seem primarily about identification, for which we now use terms such as 'community' or 'neighbourhood'. How might such concepts be embedded in the design and layout of a new community, suburb or even a new town? It is of interest that the core of the new 'neighbourhood units' proposed by the American Clarence Perry in 1929, by Lord Reith's New Towns Committee in 1945 and in Patrick Abercrombie's 1944 plans for 11 new neighbourhoods in the war-torn East End of London was the catchment area for a junior school. This was a unit of upwards of 6,000 people in which no child should have to cross a main road to get to school (Harwood and Powers 2001, 142). These new secular 'tribal' territories thus took over the topographical role once held by the urban Christian parish. However, since not all the inhabitants were directly involved with the school once the children had left, that central building was not as dominant a tribal focus as the medieval church once was. That said, in the 21st century, many urban residents identify rather more with the various cultural tribes they interact with (be it their work colleagues, faith group, football supporters' club or whatever) than with the postcode where they currently reside.

The tribe-sized nature of human societies has been discussed by Professor Dunbar in the social brain hypothesis: this was the result of a study of brain size (the neocortex) and evolutionary social interactions (Dunbar 1998). He suggested that the 'natural' group size for humans is about 150, which is three times larger than most of the more social apes, a consequence of the social use of music and, later, language. This number seems to be reflected not only in the typical size of small-scale hunter-gatherer societies, but also "in personal social networks in contemporary society as well as in the modal number of friends listed on Facebook pages" (Dunbar 2014, 109). He goes on to suggest that our social networks could be structured in concentric circles, in which the central 150 circle defines our key bilateral relationships, those that come with obligations and reciprocity. An outer circle of a further 500 might include all those we would call acquaintances (known to us but with fewer obligations), while the outermost ring of up to 1,500 represents all those faces we could put a name to, whether friends or not (Dunbar 2014, 11, fig. 2).

It could be argued that social interactions and recognition in an urban situation are a little more complex than that. Indeed, it seems that as societies grew more complex in their structure, so too did the languages required to facilitate them. In a major conurbation, we are obliged to be members of more than one tribe at a time, and thus for some of the more influential social groupings (tribes) with which we must identify, each one may have its own 150-person centre and its attendant penumbra. In other words, rather than one single core with ever widening outer circuits, we inhabit perhaps as many as four, five or more overlapping (but smaller) circular tribes. Thus the evolutionary determinants of the size of our modern social groupings have been culturally adapted and developed to enable us to cope with urban populations. This modular mental restructuring (polytribalisation) is nevertheless still based on the effective size of those ancient hunter-gatherer groups. The implications for the most efficient organisation of businesses, the civil service, schools and call centres need further detailed study in the light of this evolutionary concept. As E. F. Schumacher suggested in his book *Small is Beautiful* (1973), to work with maximum effect, large corporations and similar organisations need to operate like a series of related sub-groups, or 'tribes' in evolutionary-determinant terminology.

But the complexity of modern urban society is not just multi-tribal, since it is also increasingly multi-layered. There are the tribes we willingly identify ourselves with, and then there are those that other people identify us with, to which we become unwilling members. The occupational tribes we belong to can and do change over time, but residual allegiances may remain; although we may wish it otherwise, we move between age-related tribes, eventually being promoted to the senior citizenry. Some tribes are property related or income related, both of which can and do change over time, and not always in the right direction. Our cultural, political and religious affiliations may also alter, perhaps as we change our geography, postcode, employment, age or circumstances. Modern cities are therefore structured socially in a most complex and ever-changing way; it is not the most logical of systems, since our social brain, while certainly capable of adapting to new challenges, is still programmed with a tribal-sized Palaeolithic default. This has implications for the concepts of 'community' and 'neighbourhood' as used and misused by politicians and town planners, since these usually seem to refer to postcodes rather than the subtle and complex polytribal social environment within which the rest of the population live.

Hunter–gatherers in the modern city

Those who work in HR departments, and thus review many CVs on a daily basis, will be aware that the basic hunter-type and the basic gatherer-type are still very much present in the modern city. The first is an acknowledged team player, but able to work on their own initiative when required, is up for a challenge and has a strong love of sports (including the extreme ones). The second is happy to provide a reliable and responsible support role, is highly organised, with a strong attention to detail, and likes walking and gardening. Those Palaeolithic drives and imperatives that underpin hunting and gathering have not been extinguished, but they have been redirected over time into proxy activities, of which the most obvious are football and shopping.

To return to medieval London, few citizens would have had the time to comb the hedgerows checking to see where the new shoots were and which fruits, nuts or roots were already ripe. This would have required a daily group excursion into the green belt. Instead, the produce of the surrounding countryside was brought to them, and thus Londoners could make their selections in the marketplace, rather than in wide open spaces, while still retaining the important social focus of such gathering activities; after all, harvesting nature in the Palaeolithic was as much about education and social bonding as it was about finding food. Thus such markets became an important social focus. Shopping for some is now more about fashion than food. But even then, in its most modern and most urbane guise of retail therapy, the food-gatherers' vocabulary of colour and seasonality (the autumn collection) lingers on. It's just that we have exchanged 'ripe' for 'on trend' and the potentially fatal 'over-ripe' for 'so last year'.

The need to set up a store of food against harder times also remains with us, but manifests itself in the universal drive to collect. It seems to be still embedded in male and female, adult and child, and is reflected in everything from lists of train numbers to first editions, autographs, shoes, handbags, militaria, fine wines, souvenirs, football programmes, jewellery, CDs, ties, postcards, bottles, conkers and figurines. It's a universal habit that the invention of the deep-freeze and the 24-hour supermarket should have solved, but the drive is so strong that we have transferred its energies and focus from food to consumer durables and any manner of collectables.

Being a collector is not in itself considered antisocial behaviour, but the same psychological process or primeval drive can have some unwelcome manifestations in modern society, in the form of, for example, kleptomania and obsessive hoarding. Kleptomania is a psychiatric disorder that involves an uncontrollable urge to take things, but differs from standard theft in that the items are not stolen for personal use or for their intrinsic monetary value. Although such thefts are sometimes associated with substance abuse, they are not concerned with antagonism or revenge, and they are not a reaction to delusions or fantasies. Some individuals with kleptomania also demonstrate hoarding symptoms that resemble those with obsessive compulsive disorder, and kleptomania occurs more frequently among women than men.

Perhaps significantly, those classed as kleptomaniacs are characterised by a total inability to prevent or contain the urge to take things, an escalating sense of pressure immediately before the theft and a sense of satisfaction, fulfilment or relief as the theft itself takes place. Some may recognise that particular pattern as not dissimilar to retail therapy, but with 'purchase' substituted for 'theft'. Psychoanalytic theorists suggest that kleptomania is a person's attempt "to obtain symbolic compensation for an actual or anticipated loss" (Cupchik and Atcheson 1983, 350); it is suggested here, however, that, like compulsive hoarding, it's a perversion of the once dominant force that drove the hunter-gatherer to collect enough fruit, berries, plants or nuts each day, every day just to survive. It may be the 21st century for us, but that's not necessarily the case for our Palaeolithic genome.

To take another example: compulsive hoarding, or hoarding disorder, is characterised by the excessive collection of large quantities of objects which overfill the home, coupled with an inability or unwillingness to discard any of the items. In its worst manifestations, compulsive hoarding can cause fires, rodent or roach infestations and other health and safety hazards. It seems to be becoming increasingly common, and prevalence rates have been estimated at nearly 4%, but are greater in men than women (Samuels et al. 2008). The condition typically manifests in childhood, with symptoms worsening with advancing age. Hoarding behaviour is often so severe because the hoarders do not recognise it as a problem, but see it as perfectly natural. In a Palaeolithic context, hoarding was in fact just that: perfectly natural. Understanding the deeply immersed rationale for such antisocial behaviour is not to excuse the acts, but to help provide a reasoned response and a possible cure, or suggest an aversion therapy or an effective substitute behaviour.

Violence is on our bones

The Seville Statement on Violence was signed in 1986 by a group of scientists with the best of intentions. It stated that war or other violent behaviour was not genetically programmed into our nature. Those who study human evolution, however, might argue that the capacity to be an effective hunter remains in our genes, and this inherited attribute can still result in violent and highly antisocial behaviour. It is not, of course, inevitable. The real question is how that disposition is used or abused in our modern context, since there is rarely a genuine imperative to kill to survive, at least not in this town or in this decade.

Violence by humans towards animals being hunted for food must have a long history; conflict between human groups, by contrast, was once thought to be a more recent development. It was widely considered as a direct consequence of the Agricultural Revolution, the movement that required fixed territories to be laid out and 'permanent' settlements to be established. Given that previously the landscape had been open and devoid of proprietary borders, the new regime would have demanded that the new farms and settlements be protected against 'outsiders'. In such situations, conflict over land ownership and resources would ultimately become inevitable as populations grew and the demand for food grew with them.

Evidence that violence by humans on humans has a regrettably longer history than that is slowly emerging from sites such as Nataruk in Turkana County, Kenya. This site has been dated to about 10,000 BP, well before the farming revolution reached this part of the continent. Recent investigations have revealed the remains of 21 adults and six children all of whom had met a violent death. Two of the adult males had stone projectile tips lodged in the skull and throat, while other skeletons show lesions in the head, neck, ribs, hands and knees caused by clubs or wooden-handled weapons with hafted sharp stone blades that caused deep cuts. Two individuals, including a young woman who was heavily pregnant at the time, had no lesions in the preserved parts of the skeleton, but the position of their hands suggests they may have been bound. The bodies were left unburied in what was once the shallow waters of a lake, now long since dried up.

This region at that time was fertile, providing plenty of fish, game and plant produce. There are fossil remains of elephants, hippos, rhinos, giraffes, zebras, warthogs, buffalos, antelopes, gazelles, primates, hyraxes, snakes, turtles and crocodiles, as well as lions, hyenas and wild dogs. Compared to the immediately surrounding areas, the freshwater lake with its open shoreline provided the best and richest hunting grounds for many miles. The archaeologists Dr Marta Mirazón Lahr and her colleagues (2016) have suggested that it was the very abundance of resources in this particular location which led to the death of the Nataruk hunter-gathering group. Whether the killing field represents a new group straying into the territory of an established community, or whether an established community was dispatched by aggressive new arrivals is less certain; what is clear is that such a richly resourced site was deemed worth fighting for, and the hunters became the hunted.

The ability to track and kill a wild animal requires the same skills and mindset as those needed to kill human intruders, if they threaten your own survival. But simply having the capacity for violence is no excuse for being unnecessarily violent, since today such uncivilised drives can be readily and constructively channelled into rather more socially acceptable urban activities.

Nimrod variations

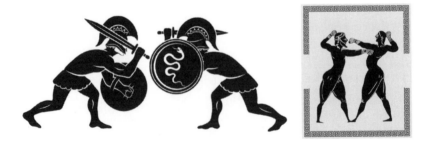

Figure 9.1. *Plus ça change?* Ancient Greece: hand-to-hand combat in war (left) and sporting boxers in peace time (right).

To return to the hunting psyche and its continuing relationship with urbanisation: initially, London's medieval citizens retained the right to hunt in the woodlands that still surrounded the capital, in Middlesex, Hertfordshire, Kent and the Chilterns. In the late 12th century, this pastime usually involved dogs or birds, such as merlins or hawks, and provided game for the table (Wheatley 1956, 509). Sports of various levels of physicality had also been developed as a proxy for hunting and military prowess. Events included leaping, wrestling, archery, javelin and stone-throwing or fighting with bucklers. As the contemporary commentator William Fitzstephen noted in 1170, "Youth is an age eager for glory and delirious of victory, and so young men engage in counterfeit battles so that they conduct themselves more valiantly in real ones" (Wheatley 1956, 509: a line written before the playing fields of Eton had been laid out).

We also learn that at Whitsuntide, "after dinner all the young men of the (medieval) City go out into the fields to play at the well-known game of football. The scholars belonging to the several schools have each their ball: and the City tradesmen, according to their respective crafts, have theirs. The more aged men, the fathers of the players and the wealthy citizens, come on horseback to see the contests … their natural heat seeming to be aroused by the sight of so much agility" (Wheatley 1956, 507). In such ways, the City's various tribal identities were made manifest, the citizenry engaged in daily exercise and channelled their well-honed hunting abilities into socially acceptable physical violence.

How such deep drives are utilised in a modern urban society is a complex question. In urban life, the hunting mentality re-emerges in various guises, not just in military service. For many, there are genre computer games that provide an outlet for hunting and killing, albeit more or less cerebral and, in terms of environment, far removed from the wide open African savannah. The provision of such sedentary proxy-hunting is big business (according to the BBC, *Call of Duty* sold 2.7 million copies in the UK in 2012), requires considerable technical skill and creativity to resource, and keeps adolescents of all ages (and genders) absorbed for hours. In a bizarre perversion of life, there is now an electronic sports league (ESL) in which four million players compete with each other as they roam across cyberspace, responding to the ancient evolutionary need to hunt and kill while sitting comfortably indoors.

The most obvious modern substitute for the hunt is active sport, combining as it does physical exertion, teamwork and adrenalin with the prospect of personal and social reward. Many team sports, developed by different agencies at different times, naturally utilise similar sized groupings to the ancient hunting parties. Even the rather larger fifteen-person rugby union team employs a smaller eight-man sub-unit, rather significantly termed a 'pack'. And football, whether at the level of a local pub team, a parish or the Premier League, has tribe and territory written through and through it. The deep origin of such sports is not hard to see; the surprise is rather how persistent and prolonged the need has remained, and how urgently each new generation demands that it be satisfied. We have not as yet grown out of the habit of pretending to hunt.

There are consequently many modern manifestations of the hunting psyche, some less socially desirable than others. In the West there are many who fish as a recreational activity rather than as a survival strategy. From William the Conqueror onwards, the English king and his knights saw hunting as their prerogative, establishing vast chases or forests as their exclusive hunting grounds. For them, warriors and hunters were one and the same. As for the lower orders, they were not called hunters but poachers, and punished accordingly. Interestingly, in the UK (but not in the US) the relationship between hunting and the social elite remains strong. Here, hunting for some has been transformed into corporate grouse shoots and fox-hunting cavalcades, as the ancient drive has become increasingly ritualised by some and ridiculed by others. Another attribute of the hunting mindset is the need to be challenged and to take risks; for some this can be channelled into extreme sports, for example, while for others it can involve gambling and trying your luck against the odds. Neither approach makes any rational sense, but then neither does hunting wild animals rather than picking fruit.

Crime science

It is now clear that a burglar, whether stealing from houses or cars, makes use of the same skills that an ancient hunter would have done. Sometimes the 'kill' is the result of a pre-planned and careful stake-out, sometimes an opportunistic act. Professor Jeffrey Brantingham of the University of California, Los Angeles (UCLA) studies hunter-gatherers in northern Tibet, and puts that research to use with the Los Angeles Police Department in the analysis of crime patterns. As he has elegantly stated: "Criminal offenders are essentially hunter-gatherers; they forage for opportunities to commit crimes: the behaviours that a hunter-gatherer uses to choose a wildebeest versus a gazelle are the same calculations a criminal uses to choose a Honda versus a Lexus" (Wolpert 2010; see also Shorta et al. 2010). Both activities are potentially high-risk strategies, have similar adrenalin rushes and can become addictive.

Similarly, an urban street gang is basically a modern-day perversion of a hunting group, with its powerful bonding and adherence to a very particular territory. Gang culture therefore needs to be seen not just in present-day societal terms, but its deeper roots also need to be appreciated if an effective remedy for its violent spiral is ever to be administered. In 2013, the *London Evening Standard*'s campaigns editor, David Cohen, began a ground-breaking series on the city's gangs and the climate of urban violence that surrounds them. He reported, for example, on a detailed study of over 100 children drawn from 18,000 of the most vulnerable individuals being helped by the Kids Company charity, and drew some stark conclusions. The research was conducted at UCL by Charlotte Cecil, and supervised by Professor Essi

Viding and Dr Eamon McCory. It reports that almost half had witnessed a stabbing or shooting in their own community, 25% had witnessed a murder and 20% had themselves been shot or stabbed. In addition, this was a group that was far more likely to have personally experienced physical or sexual abuse than the average London child (Cecil et al. 2014). The roots for developing an ever-increasing cycle of violence are all too clear.

That time-bomb has already begun exploding: from 2005 to 2014 there have been 185 teenage murders in London, of which 128 were stabbings (see http://www.citizensreportuk.org/reports/teenage-murder-london. html; Kinsella 2011). According to the Metropolitan Police, there are at least 250 gangs in the sprawling capital, of which 54 are considered to be the most active, being held responsible for two-thirds of the capital's gang-related crime. This challenge is being taken very seriously, with a special unit of 1,000 dedicated police officers, using a balance of enforcement and prevention: tough on crime, tough on the causes of crime, as a government spin doctor once put it. And the first results, at least in terms of lowering rates of violent crime, are encouraging.

But while the political imperative to 'break' gangs is strong, it is worth considering the evolutionary social roots which underpin them. There have been several detailed studies of gang culture, including Malcolm Klein's *The American Street Gang* (1995) and *The Eurogang Paradox* (Klein et al. 2001). A heavier police presence, softer community-based methodologies, policies of zero tolerance, knife and gun amnesties, counselling, boot camps and employment training are just some of the approaches attempted to counter this social problem, but often with no concerted effort to establish the relative long-term effectiveness of these widely contrasting methods.

Sports science

One of the most telling sentences in the work undertaken on gangs is this: "most youth join gangs, not in order to commit crime, but in order to meet personal and social needs for identity, for status, for excitement, for a sense of belonging, and for a false sense of protection" (Klein et al. 2001, 330). The first four of these needs can all be met by any form of vigorous teamwork, such as sport, one of the standard ways the hunter mindset can be constructively reconfigured. Compton, for example, is a notorious gang-infested suburb of Los Angeles, but it boasts a cricket team formed in 1995. According to the club's website (www.comptoncricketclub.us), the team was founded to fight poverty and crime with the civilising qualities of cricket. The evolutionary anthropologist would claim that it was not the cricket per se, but the basic need of males to be part of a team, to have increased self-esteem and to be fully involved in a physically demanding but exhilarating regime.

That sport can be used as a socially positive proxy for hunting (and therefore gang culture) has been ably demonstrated by the Midnight Basketball movement which started in the United States in 1986 (Hartmann and Depro 2006), and proved equally as effective in Australia, where it has operated since 2007. These programmes offer organised sport, education and personal development, discipline, social inclusion and enhanced self-esteem (rather than a life of petty crime, drugs, violence and other social problems). In London, where football is the team sport of choice, especial mention must be made of the Kickz programme. Working in inner-city schools in Islington, Hackney and Camden, the Arsenal in the Community team aims to encourage increased participation in sport, providing positive personal development in addition to a healthier lifestyle. Its wider goals include improved social cohesion as well as lowering rates of crime and drug abuse. Their project on the Elthorne Park estate, run in conjunction with the Metropolitan Police, began in 2006, following a year in which some 2,529 youth crimes were reported in the area. By 2009, that annual figure was down to just 867, a drop of 66% (Laureus 2010). It can never be proved precisely what percentage of that reduction is directly attributable to the Kickz scheme itself, but all those involved could see it was a key factor. Similar results, both anecdotal and statistically verified, can be seen with, for example, the Tottenham Boxing Academy or Jim Armstrong's Laburnum Boat Club. As one committed participant observed when asked if kayaking kept him away from gangs: "it's kept them away from me" (Cohen 2016).

While the social success of such schemes can be amply justified by their results, the underlying reasons for their effectiveness are not, as yet, fully understood. A better understanding of the evolutionary determinants of social behaviour provides a window that looks beyond the current cultural and social complexities. It could help to ensure that the new initiatives can be extended more effectively, and that clear directions are provided to facilitate and encourage the necessary changes in coherent and integrated public policy programmes. Crime science, sports science, social workers, the Metropolitan Police and London's youth could all benefit from such an approach. It is significant that the Arsenal in the Community team are now experimenting with a new approach to gang members: rather than trying to break up the gangs, they are trying to accommodate the whole unit. They are accepting them as one of 'our gangs', and then encouraging them en bloc to focus their energies on less antisocial activities. If this enlightened approach proves effective, then it will be another example of how going with the grain and working with our ancient drives might offer dividends.

To widen the debate on the evolutionary link between hunting, aggression, violence and sport: if sport can have a beneficial role to play in an urban context, might it also carry some weight on the global stage? The Christmas Truce on the Western Front during the First World War has become legendary: front-line troops from the opposing German and British infantry divisions, having sung festive carols, then cautiously met up in the no-man's land that separated the trenches. The bodies of dead comrades were retrieved, souvenirs were exchanged and, most famously, a game of football was played. Could wars really be decided on a playing field? The upper echelons of the military machine thought not, and frowned on such fraternisation, working assiduously to stamp it out. But if one small kick-about could delay the killing for a day on one small section of the front line, what might a proper tournament do? For my generation, we didn't think the Second World War was really all over until after Geoff Hurst's Wembley hat-trick in the 4-2 win against Germany in July 1966. Interestingly, the Russian linesman, when asked why he awarded the controversial third goal to England, is said to have muttered, "Stalingrad", while the English fans then began the chant, "Two world wars and one World Cup". Sport and war were (and are) closely linked in the collective subconscious.

Indeed, there is an obvious correlation between wars and years in which the Olympic Games were not held or boycotted (e.g. 1916 (First World War), 1940 and 1944 (Second World War), 1956 (Suez/Hungary), 1980 (Afghanistan)). If you were from Mars, it could therefore be suggested that the Games (and indeed the FIFA World Cup) were an either/or substitute for international aggression. You could have a world war or you could have a World Cup, but you can't have both. The need to participate in competitive sports meets the same basic evolutionary drive that underpins the hunter/warrior psyche: if we had more international sport, would we therefore have fewer international wars? Or would we ever see a truce declared to let the Games begin? I would doubt that in my lifetime, but it might just provide a rationale for a revived League of Nations.

Meanwhile, back in London, the opportunity to capitalise on the Olympic legacy of 2012 and 2016 needs no stressing. There is currently a political incentive to make an 'investment in sport', but how effective such a programme will prove to be in the long run – in terms of much increased levels of physical activity and social cohesion at all levels of society – remains to be seen. Would a chronically obese nation sitting on its collective sofa watching Team GB win an even greater haul of gold medals in Tokyo in 2020 be seen as a success? Surely, it is at the level of each and every school that the real story must begin, with the work of projects such as those pioneered by the Arsenal in the Community team. But unless there are playing fields and sports facilities provided in the neighbourhood, and unless there is a culture that promotes their use, then the full personal, social and health benefits might not be realised. The provision of places where physical activities can take place at team, family and personal levels takes us back, once again, to town planning issues. The larger the conurbation, the greater the need for readily accessible sports halls, playing fields, swimming baths, large parks, cycle tracks and safe, car-free pedestrianised areas. Such evolutionary-concordant infrastructure simultaneously promotes both active lifestyles and social cohesion.

Chapter 10

MUSIC AND WORDS

Darwin claims that the power of producing and appreciating [music] existed among the human race long before the power of speech was arrived at. Perhaps that is why we are so subtly influenced by it. There are vague memories in our souls in those misty centuries when the world was in its childhood.

Arthur Conan Doyle (1859–1930)

On song

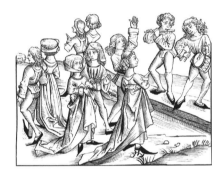 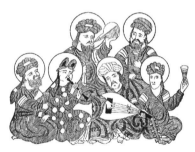

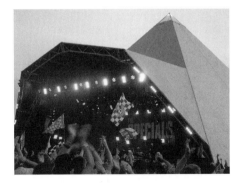

Figure 10.1. Hymns ancient and modern: music played an important social role in the past as this medieval image shows (left), and is certainly universal (right). As at Glastonbury Festival, it still has the power to unite and move us.

The animal kingdom is full of the sound of music: even in the middle of town, we have all heard pigeons cooing in the springtime, the piercing alarm call of blackbirds, dogs barking to defend their territory and cats purring in contentment. Simple sounds can therefore convey the strongest message, stripped of ambiguity. And we all seem to share an understanding of music in some form. The psychobiologist Harry Witchel has argued that one of music's key roles is in establishing human territory, in terms of our varied social identities (Witchel 2011).

As for music's role in the mating game across the animal kingdom, the study of this has a long history. Charles Darwin, for example, noted that amphibians such as frogs and toads "possess vocal chords which are incessantly used during the breeding season". At such a time, the male tortoise might be heard, as well as the roar of the alligator. He then goes on to discuss the differing vocal abilities of mammals, male and female, with particular regard to primates (Darwin 1871, 633–634).

As for the modern human race, while accepting the cultural diversity of 'music', its very universality clearly argues for a deep common origin (see e.g. Blacking 1973; Wallin et al. 2000). It is argued here that we could sing long, long before we could speak: music is an essential part of our Palaeolithic inheritance. For any ancient society to function, there had to be communication between individuals, between individuals and families, between working groups and the tribe as a whole. It has been proposed that to establish when, in our long evolutionary journey, we finally gained the power of speech would be to establish when we became truly human. But recent research suggests that before we could talk, we had to learn to sing, and thus it was music that made us human.

Language, whether written, spoken, emailed or texted, has become the cornerstone of human communication. Without this relatively new-found ability to communicate complex detailed information (or indeed trivial gossip), 'civilisation' – as we know it – could not have developed or expanded. Although pets might appear to understand every word we say, and parrots might accurately mimic choice phrases, our highly sophisticated verbal communication system was an invention by *Homo sapiens* for *Homo sapiens*, the product (or progenitor?) of increasing human brain power in the Palaeolithic period. But what was life like for our earliest ancestors in a world devoid of words? What systems did the early hunter-gatherers use to communicate before articulate speech? What might be the relationship between the old and the new systems? And what happened to those pre-language languages once words became commonplace and took on a life of their own? The prehistoric system seems to have been a varied one including utterances such as laughter or threats, body language and eye contact, sign language and gesturing, outward displays of emotion and rhythmic or melodic communication. All these elements were, and indeed still can be, used independently or in concert.

Half a million years ago, it seems we still depended on body language and sign language and, for want of a better term, 'music'. It was those systems, not unrelated, that provided communication, information and much more. Our version of body language, which in general terms is shared by many others in the animal kingdom, has a rich repertoire. Smiles, scowls, eye contact, waving, fists, hand holding, I-need-a-hug, blushing, crying: all are intended to send or receive messages, voluntarily or involuntarily. And we are not just good at gesturing, for we can also mimic or copy what we see, and thus can develop complex sign languages. We have never lost our ability to access these systems of connection and communication, in spite of our ever-expanding vocabularies; indeed, we are adding new 'words' to the more ancient system with hand signals such as Churchill's 'victory' sign, 'phone me' and the internationally understood gesture for 'May I have the bill, please?' As for the actual words we use in everyday speech, it's often the way they are said and the body language that accompanies them that carries the strongest message. Similarly, if we choose to communicate with babies or pets using the Queen's English, although the facts will be lost in transmission, the meaning will not.

There is, of course, a strong relationship between music and body language: dancing, clapping, chanting and many children's games all integrate the two systems. So too do marching and working songs, spurred on by the rhythms of bipedalism and repetitive actions (how ancient must they be?). But what is the relationship of music to language, that rather more complex mode of social and personal communication? It has long been supposed that 'speech makes man', setting that particular creature apart from the rest of nature. Writing a century before Darwin, the papers published between 1773 and 1792 by James Burnett (Lord Monboddo) were among the first to develop this concept of 'the origin and progress of language'.

Whereas Dr Blackstock proposed that "the first language among men was music, and that before our ideas were expressed by articulate sounds, they were communicated by tones, varied in different degrees of gravity and acuteness" (Darwin 1871, 639). Charles Darwin himself agreed and advanced the following argument:

---

as we have every reason to suppose that articulate speech is one of the latest, as it certainly is the highest, of the arts acquired by man, and as the instinctive power of producing musical notes and rhythms is developed low down in the animal series, it would be altogether opposed to the principle of evolution if we were to admit that man's musical capacity has been developed from the tones used in impassioned speech. We must assume that the rhythms and cadences of oratory are derived from previously developed musical powers. We can thus understand that music, dancing, song and poetry are such ancient arts. We may go even further than this and … believe that musical sounds afforded one of the bases for the development of language. (Darwin 1871, 638–639)

The challenge of converting Darwin's belief into demonstrable facts over the next 150 years has been admirably summarised by Nicholas Bannan in a multi-disciplinary study that combines human evolution, linguistics, biolinguistics, social and cognitive psychology, musicology, animal behaviour and neuroscience, to name some of the avenues explored (2012a). Although Pinker, in *How the Mind Works* (1997), could find no sensible use or function for music in human evolution, almost everyone else who has studied this concept suggests that it could have played a key role in sexual selection, group cohesion and information transfer (Foley 2012, 50).

Archaeologists have recovered musical instruments which are at least 35,000 years old (Bannan 2012b, 14), so music might be substantially older than that, and substantially older than our ability to articulate words. The last common ancestor shared by chimpanzees and humans lived some six to seven million years ago. It seems that neither that creature nor the subsequent line of chimpanzees that descended from it could ever sing; musicality must therefore be an acquired attribute unique to the human branch. Indeed, given the universality of musical abilities in all modern human populations, it must have a solid genetic basis that must have been in place at least 200,000 years ago (Foley 2012, 35–49).

The long-running debate on the relationship of singing to speaking, and whether musicality pre-dates language, continues, but there is increasing evidence to support this proposition. Evolutionary psychologists, such as Professor Robin Dunbar (2012), for example, accept that music did have a central role in the development of language, since it seems to have replaced grooming as the principal bonding mechanism for the evolving human primates. It has been suggested that 'language' developed in at least three phases, of which the first was represented by physical body language, which included the grooming process during which primates carefully picked out fleas and smoothed the coats of their fellows. Who was allowed to groom whom dictated the complex personal and social relationships. Some 500,000 years ago, some of the social aspects of grooming may have been superseded by the second phase, wordless vocal exchanges or 'chorusing' (although how this affected the fleas is not explained).

Evolutionary determinants of music

Anatomically, this could well reflect the dramatic expansion of the vertebral column in the thoracic region, together with an increase in size of the hypoglossal nerve: these evolutionary developments would have respectively improved breath control as well as control of the tongue, greatly facilitating vocalisation (Dunbar 2012, 208–209). However, it seems as though the FOXP2 gene, which is regarded as essential for the evolution of full grammatical language, did not appear until some 200,000 years ago, with the arrival of modern *Homo sapiens*. Since singing requires the same levels of voice control as speech, it could thus be argued that forms of singing held sway for perhaps 300,000 years before the same physiological attributes that facilitated wordless singing were subsequently used for articulating musicless words (Dunbar 2012, 209–210).

Also working from the perspective of the evolution of the human vocal tract, Margaret Clegg (Natural History Museum) suggests that our ability to speak "developed from our existing anatomy and capabilities. Humans sound the way they do by accident, not design. The anatomy of the vocal tract that allows us to produce the sounds of speech is fortuitous, and not a necessary prerequisite" (Clegg 2012, 73–74). Taken together, it could thus be argued that singing (or chorusing) was the preferred mode of communication among early humans for far longer than speech has been; quite enough time to develop complex skills and accomplished techniques in this field. These and other fascinating insights were discussed at a major conference held in Reading in 2004, now published as a major volume that explores the development of music, language and human evolution (Bannan 2012a).

The following year, archaeologist Steven Mithen (University of Reading) argued that "we can only explain the human propensity to make and listen to music by recognising that is has been encoded into the human genome during the evolutionary history of our species" (Mithen 2005, 1). His book, *The Singing Neanderthals*, then goes on to suggest how, when and why this happened. He expands on the subtle interrelationship between 'music' and language as we know it today, and then to 'musilanguage', the common root of both systems suggested by Steven Brown (2000), as well as the holistic proto-language proposed by Alison Wray (2000a, 2000b, 2002). Mithen proposes his own term for a pre-language sub-language, 'Hmmmmm' (Mithen 2005, 172), an acronym for holistic, manipulative, multi-modal, musical and mimetic. That list – a fusion of body language and music – embodies many of the necessary components in which sounds and actions can be combined to convey various levels of information.

He goes on to suggest that Hmmmmm, his musical proto-language, functioned effectively enough in the milieu of socially uncomplex, small-scale hunter-gathering societies. But the development of larger-scale civilisations with more complex economies and social hierarchies demanded a greater facility and ability to communicate ever more elaborate information. His thesis is thus that a form of music was our first means of social communication. In this, it seems that there is now a consensus building. However, Mithen then suggests that the musical proto-language was superseded by grammatical 'language' (the now all-powerful written or spoken word) as society became more complex. He argues that music was subsequently rather relegated to a cultural sideline, developing as an entertainment or vehicle for religious or emotional expression.

Potency of music

But did words really supersede music? Arguably, the relatively modern development of a complex feature such as language should be seen as an addition to our armoury, rather than a straight substitution of new for old. It is of some interest to see and hear the way that children mix music, rhythm and verse (often just doggerel) in games that involve skipping, hopping and clapping, or at least this used to be the case some decades ago. Such activities were hardly poetry and only just musical, but they were certainly convivial social communicators: the words were only sounds but had purpose, if not meaning. Modern language remains the most logical way of communicating detailed information, but we have not lost our ability to tune into and utilise the more ancient musical and physical proto-languages of our distant pre-urban lives.

Indeed, why is it that politicians find the cadences of rhetorical convention a more effective means of communicating than reciting statistics? Why do advertisers use jingles, and film-makers use music to sell their products? Why do football crowds chant, nations demand anthems, religions require hymns, lovers recognise 'their song' and people on long journeys lock themselves into their iPods? All are still using the 500,000-year-old proto-language to the full: communication is not just about hard facts.

Music can therefore do many things and play many parts. Each genre provides a clear tribal identity, unmistakably delineating the common ground shared by its members. For those on their own, it provides company; it has a unique ability to store memories; and is a most dramatic social catalyst for those who enjoy communal singing, playing in orchestras, bands or groups or dancing, strictly or otherwise. In fact, its latent power as an ancient and highly effective communicator is still utilised in therapeutic practices. To give one example, the Key Changes programme has worked in Islington since 2008. It provides musical activities for some 300 patients in psychiatric hospitals in that London borough each year. Trained thera-pists and professional musicians provide music engagement and recovery services for young people and adults experiencing severe mental illnesses, including psychosis, schizophrenia, bipolar and personality disorders. For those who are less responsive to the spoken word and have difficulty engag-ing with others, music in its many forms provides a deeper means of communication and can help build a route back into wider society. Music therapy is also used effectively for children with autism, while dancing classes for the disabled have been shown to be especially beneficial. In addi-tion, Emeli Sandé, the Brit Award-winning singer, also believes in the potency of music for social change. She is visiting prisons for the Key4Life programme to inspire inmates to move from crime to careers in the music industry (Watts 2016).

That music in all its forms of rhythmic and melodic communication is so universal, and can achieve so much, is reason enough to argue for its antiquity. It must have deep, instinctive roots, certainly older than urbanism, clearly older than formal language and potentially older than humanity itself. Given such a pedigree, it should be a warmly welcomed component of an evolutionary-concordant urban life (although some draw the line at bagpipes).

Good Vibrations

The potency of music to effect short- and long-term positive behaviour change is clearly illustrated by the example of Gamelan percussion. Music sessions have been performed in many UK prisons with the hard-working charity Good Vibrations. Since 2003 they have involved 3,600 participants in over 53 secure institutions including Brixton, Holloway, Pentonville and Wandsworth in London, as well as others across the country, such as Broadmoor, Dartmoor, Garston, Rampton and Wakefield. The Indonesian style of music was selected for these activities because it is readily accessible and requires no previous musi-cal experience or an ability to read musical notation. Importantly, it is a communal activity with no conductor necessary, in which each individ-ual's contribution is equally important, since everyone has to listen to each other to fit in (Digard et al. 2007).

The following quote is taken from the Good Vibrations website (www. good-vibrations.org.uk):

Coming from lives often characterised by abuse, oppression, or lack of opportunity, an experience where each individual's opin-ions were valued had great therapeutic potential.

Increasingly, group members spontaneously and independently controlled their own behaviour, without needing prompts from more focused group members.

The sessions are recorded as having improved confidence, listening and communication skills, tolerance, social interaction (with staff as well as with other participants), levels of self-expression and the ability to cope with stress and prison life. For many, these changes were sustained in the longer term. Music's deeply embedded power is reflected in this final quote:

The Gamelan music produced by the participants carried meaning for them that they could not verbalise, or perhaps did not consciously recognise. One participant reported how she felt the music spoke to her soul and calmed her in a way she could not describe. Other participants expressed similar sentiments – that they had experienced a sensation of peace and connection that they could not do justice to through verbal description.

In terms of seeing music's evolutionary function as a pre-language means of social communication, interaction and control, these are all illuminating statements. Music was not always just an optional cultural addition to social life: it was a (perhaps the?) prime catalyst for tribal cohesion and social development, from which our later literate civilisations evolved. It still remains a powerful force in its own right, a deeper and more common communicator than mere words alone.

Chapter 11

GREEN AND PLEASANT

How fair is a garden amid the trials and passions of existence.

Benjamin Disraeli (1804–1881)

For the love of nature

Why, as we move through the increasingly urbanised and technologically sophisticated world of the 21st century, are gardening and wildlife programmes still enduringly popular themes for family entertainment on the small (or not so small) screen? And what is the connection between houseplants, parks, pets and patios? The answer is that they are all modern responses to our innate and deeply felt need to connect with or respond to what we now call Nature. That's an interesting noun, one we use to identify the world seemingly beyond our artificial environment. But to what extent should our towns be 'unnatural' or 'non-natural', and should we consider us humans as being too evolved to be regarded as mere animals any more? Perhaps a new definition of 'human nature' is required.

Many of the evolutionary determinants of health considered in this book can be related to aspects of our physiology and psychology that were present in our ancestral family at least three million years ago. Arguably there are other conditions that are even older in origin, since we have also inherited a pre-human evolutionary legacy, relating to a time when, by anybody's definition, we were still paid-up members of the animal kingdom. One such is our biophilia, those instinctive, biological connections between humans and the living world, as discussed in Edward O. Wilson's pioneering study of the subject (Wilson 1984). They seem to take us back beyond our immediate human ancestry (the genus *Homo*) to before the genetic divergence of the lineage of man from that of the chimpanzee and bonobo (the genus *Pan*) some six to seven million years ago, back to shared relations such as Proconsul. These were fruit- and plant-eating ape-like creatures living in the Miocene era, over 20 million years ago and more. For them, Nature was not a philosophic abstraction but a fundamental fact of life. Exposure to today's modern cities and to urban lifestyles may have numbed our primeval response to the natural world, but it certainly has not eradicated it. A love of nature is not just all in the mind: it's in our blood and our DNA too. In this chapter, we look at research which shows that suppressing our innate biophilia brings psychological and physiological problems, while more openly embracing elements of nature leads directly to enhanced urban wellbeing.

Escape to the country

The impoverished rural poor long to live in the town, with its promise of golden pavements, upward social mobility and new faces. The ground-down, inner-city worker, by contrast, yearns for a country cottage, fresh air and the green, green grass of a half-forgotten home. The bigger the town, the greater the need became. The inhabitants of the rapidly expanding cramped and polluted towns of the Industrial Revolution craved the fresh air and openness of the moors and fells, and longed to 'escape the vast city'. But free access to the countryside was not a public right, rather a cause to be fought for. As late as 1932, Benny Rothman helped to organise a mass trespass in the Derbyshire Peak District, in an area where major landowners had imposed restrictions. This action captured the public imagination: it was one of the catalysts that ultimately led (after a world war) to the 1951 designation of Britain's first four national parks in the Peak District, Lake District, Snowdonia and Dartmoor.

The concept is not a British one, but is international, since the first national park was set up in Yellowstone in the United States in 1872; another outside Sydney, Australia in 1879; the Rocky Mountains, Canada in 1885; and in Tongariro, New Zealand in 1887. The first national park in Latin America was in Puerto Rico in 1903, while Sweden led the way in Europe in 1909, and Africa had two by 1926 (Virunga and Kruger). Today there are some 7,000 national parks worldwide, of which the largest is in Greenland.

All these areas were large tracts of what could be termed 'natural' or 'semi-natural' landscape, although in Britain, at least, human activity had moulded and modified them over many generations. Nevertheless, although not necessarily a primeval wilderness, such wide open spaces were a welcome antidote to cramped city life. They were set aside from modern redevelopment to protect wildlife and promote human recreation and enjoyment. As fast as it was urbanising, the 20th century was simultaneously returning to its rural roots, and by 2010 some 15 such parks had been established in the UK. Such extensive landscapes and farmscapes provide inviting greenscape to which urban populations have welcome access. It is also accepted that living next to 'bluespace' – the seaside, rivers, lakes and canals – is also beneficial, as a recent study by Professor Mathew White's team has suggested. Working initially from the English population census data, a longitudinal panel survey showed that individuals living close to the coast reported significantly better general health and lower levels of mental health problems (White et al. 2013a, 97–103).

Even though we had rich entertainments and diverse diversions in our towns, the need to connect with an ancient landscape still remained. Perhaps, like swallows or salmon determined to return to the place of their birth, modern *Homo sapiens* still dream of their Garden of Eden. Such dreams lie behind the Wilderness Foundation UK, established in 1974 by the explorer Sir Laurens van der Post and the conservationist Dr Ian Player. The organisation works closely with the United States' WILD Foundation and South Africa's Wilderness Foundation, and is a founder member of the Wilderness Network. Not only a conservation movement, they are just as concerned with re-engaging urban populations with the natural world in its more pristine form and exploring both the spiritual and socially therapeutic dimensions of such a relationship. Their work with disturbed youngsters has measurably boosted self-esteem, decreased depression and increased levels of personal responsibility through social interaction in wilderness programmes.

Working with sometimes rather more tamed but nonetheless engaging environments, the National Trust Act 1907 ensured that particular British landscapes and buildings "of beauty or historic interest" could be preserved in perpetuity on behalf of the nation. The three founders of the National Trust were Sir Robert Hunter, Canon Hardwicke Rawnsley and Octavia Hill. The latter will also be remembered in London for her championing of social housing schemes that, by 1874, were providing decent accommodation for some 3,000 of the City's deserving poor. She also fought to protect urban greenspace, or "open air sitting rooms" as she called them. As a result of her campaigns, Londoners can still enjoy the delights of Vauxhall Park and Parliament Hill, both untrammelled by urban encroachment. Her interlinked approach to towns, nature and society was therefore one that is shared wholeheartedly by those advocating progress in town planning from a human evolutionary perspective, although she neither knew nor required those particular terms.

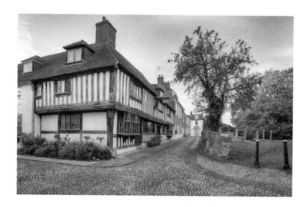

Figure 11.1. Trees and townscapes: timber buildings built from local woodlands.

Greened city: a gentle rewilding

The demands of our ancient genome vs. our contemporary urban culture are in many ways a radical revision of the long-running nature/nurture debate. In urban planning terms, this also has echoes of the equally long-running town vs. country question, in which those two features were also once positioned as contradictory opposites. Essential progress in this urban design field requires a clearer understanding of how and why the fertile middle ground represented by a green (or at least a greened) town has so much to commend it. Such a city is not so much a compromise but a desirable entity in its own right. This is not a demand for replicating nature, rewilding landscapes and simulating an untouched wilderness or a pastoral idyll. It is a more subtle compromise: the development of a modern urban settlement that has a positive relationship with nature based on an acute understanding of why we have a specific need to engage with it. That need is a key evolutionary determinant, not just for the benefit of our physical and psychological health, but also for the effective functioning of our immune systems. This chapter will discuss these three closely interlinked issues of urban wellbeing, as reflected in the challenge of introducing the natural world into that most artificial of environments, the modern city. It is a study of urban greenspace and its younger, more modest relation, urban greened space, using London as a test bed, but with diversions into the wider world as required.

One of the key evolutionary determinants of our psychological and physical health is how we react and engage with the natural world. Nature is not just an inert commodity, but a force we are obliged to interact with, as individuals and as part of urban architecture. It's the weather, it's the seasons, it's the flora, it's the fauna. Humans are not the only species to have abandoned the wide open spaces required by their hunting ancestors and adopted an urban lifestyle. So too have foxes, seagulls and magpies, to name but a few of our new city neighbours. Once we battled with carnivorous predators; now gardeners pit their wits against weeds, slugs and snails. We love robins and blackbirds, and always feed the ducks, but those responsible for the upkeep of civic buildings are less charitable with regard to pigeons. We build boxes for bats and put out nuts for birds, but poison for rats. Trees grow and keep growing: their roots can undermine our houses and their branches can block out light and buffet buses. Living by a river or next to the sea is an attractive proposition, until the flood water rises too high or storms batter the coast. A modern town cannot stand apart from nature: living with it is a two-way street.

Health and garden cities

Dr Norman Macfadyen (1877–1959) was the first medical officer of health in the new Letchworth Garden City (Hertfordshire), and a keen and distinguished promoter of that urban movement. In his passionate and compassionate pamphlet, *Health and Garden Cities*, first published in 1938, he provides data collected from the previous five years comparing health issues in the designated slum clearance areas of Manchester with the new garden satellite town of Wythenshawe.

Table 11.1. From slum to garden city

	Manchester	Wythenshawe
Infant mortality per 1,000 births	120	60
Deaths from tuberculosis per 1,000 people	1.04	0.72
Deaths from measles per 1,000 people	0.35	0.05
Deaths from influenza per 1,000 people	0.41	0.25
Deaths from bronchitis per 1,000 people	1.56	0.11
Deaths from pneumonia per 1,000 people	2.21	0.61

Source: Macfadyen 2013 [1938].

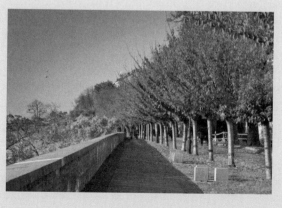

Greened city: a park in central Budapest.

Faced with such figures, there can be no denying that the greener settlement seems to offer much the better environment, and the implications for the general day-to-day health of the respective populations are obvious. That said, was it down to the greenery, the better standard of housing or the better sanitation systems in the new town?

- If it was the greenery, was it the trees, the parks, the gardens, or was it the amount of greenery, the size and extent of the greenspace, that provided the key factor?

- How important was the green belt, vis-à-vis the intramural parkland?

- What is the minimum width a green belt needs to be to function as an effective agent of health promotion?

- What is the minimum ratio of persons to acres of urban greenspace that an urban authority needs in order to convert a Manchester slum zone into a healthier settlement with the lower mortality figures in Norman Macfadyen's right-hand column?

Our ancestors relied on their natural environment and thus instinctively paid close attention to it, since their lives were lived (or lost) in the great outdoors. Even as rational city dwellers today, we have not outgrown our basic responses to the natural world. A town with a high-density population is made more bearable by having a park, for example; it is not just the size of the open space devoid of buildings and traffic noise that engages us, but the grass and trees themselves. Such a concept is hardly novel, and underlies the thinking behind Frederick Law Olmsted's Central Park in New York and Baron Haussmann's boulevards in Paris. It also underpins the garden city movement established by Sir Ebenezer Howard in 1898. He advocated socially well-ordered town plans that embraced public parks, open spaces and tree-lined streets separating industrial zones from residential areas, and with the settlement core surrounded by a green belt (Howard 1902). Howard claimed his inspiration was the utopian novel, *Looking Backward*, by Edward Bellamy (1888). With hindsight, however, it can now be appreciated at a deeper level as town planning on broadly Palaeolithic principles, confirming a basic need for 'tribal' or neighbourhood units to maintain a strong and obvious relationship with a fertile landscape.

The theory, concepts and practice of town planning have seen many changes since Howard wrote his treatise. Many would argue that a large city cannot afford to allocate the space required for the standard gardened house in a garden city: a rather greater population density is demanded for the footprint of contemporary cities. Nevertheless, a noticeable feature in today's town planners' portfolio is the heightened profile given to urban greenspace. While the development of new 'garden cities' based slavishly on Howard's visionary model are being questioned as a universal, practical option for today's urban developments, the building of a greened medium-density town is moving centre stage. It is this concept, the 'greened city', that will be discussed and expanded upon both in this chapter and the next. How much green does a town need, and what format should the greening take – one large central park or many smaller squares and pockets? But, first, the evidence on which the need for urban greenspace and urban wellbeing must be presented, which leads to the second, deeper question: why should urban greenspace be good for us?

Park life

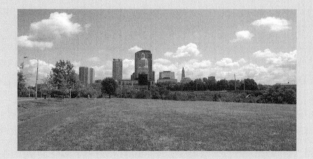

Tower blocks and urban greenspace.

A study undertaken in the city of Kaunas, Lithuania explored the relationship between the occurrence of heart disease in the population, how far people's homes were from parks and the use they made of that greenspace. It concluded that promoting increased use of urban parks could produce significant cardiovascular benefits. Between 2006 and 2008, a random sample of 5,112 people aged 45–72 was screened, and in the four-year follow-up survey there were 83 deaths from cardiovascular disease and 364 non-fatal cases of cardiovascular disease among the sampled population who had initially been free from such conditions and stroke when the study began (Tamosiunas et al. 2014). The survey and its follow-up study found:

● Increased risk of non-fatal and fatal cardiovascular disease observed for those living more than 600 m from greenspaces (hazard ratio (HR) = 1.36).

- Increased risk for non-fatal cardiovascular disease for those who were not park users and lived more than 350 m from greenspace (HR = 1.66) compared to those who lived 350 m or less from greenspace.

- Men living furthest away from parks had a higher risk of non-fatal and fatal cardiovascular disease combined, compared to those living 350 m or less from parks (HR = 1.51).

- Women who were not park users and lived 350 m or more from parks had a statistically significantly increased risk of non-fatal cardiovascular disease compared to park users living less than 350 m from parks (HR = 2.78).

- Significantly lower prevalence of cardiovascular risk factors among park users than among non-park users.

- Significantly lower prevalence of diabetes mellitus among park users than among non-park users.

Greened city: physical and psychological landscapes

There is evidence to suggest that towns are bad for us, or at least that urbanisation can lead to rising rates of psychosis and depression, according to a study published over a decade ago (Sundquist et al. 2004). Professor Mathew White from the University of Exeter is one of a number of scholars who have discussed the possibility that part of this problem may relate to the "detachment from the kinds of natural environments people evolved in and are best adapted to" (White et al. 2013b, 1). He makes reference to studies, such as one from the Netherlands, where greater levels of depression and anxiety were reported by those living in urban areas with less greenspace, in comparison with those who lived much closer to parks (Maas et al. 2009). His own study explored this question in more depth. He made use of data from 10,000 individuals recorded in the British Household Panel Survey (1991–2008) to investigate the relationship of urban greenspace to wellbeing on the one hand, and to mental distress on the other. The proximity to urban greenspace was calculated on information collected in the Generalised Land Use Database (GLUD) for England, while all the people selected were living in urban areas. The analysis of this large sample suggested that individuals felt a greater sense of wellbeing in urban areas with more greenspace. Conversely, those who lived in the less greened areas showed significantly higher levels of mental distress as well as lower life satisfaction ratings. He concluded that marked aggregate health benefits can be gained by "increasing the amount of greenspace in urban settings" (White et al. 2013a, 8,

2013b). But might that conclusion just be a reflection of the fact that richer, healthier people live in the better off greener areas, and that it was income, rather than greenspace, that was the prime agency behind the results?

A recent example from London seems to support that interpretation. The greenest and most prosperous borough is Richmond, set in the south-west of the conurbation and spanning both banks of the tree-lined Thames. In 2012, the unemployment rate was 4%, the life expectancy for women was 86 years and for men 81.5 years. For Tower Hamlets, a far greyer and more crowded inner-city borough with an unemployment rate of 13.4%, the expectancies are four to five years lower. The figures calculated for how many of those years can be considered as 'healthy' (i.e. without debilitating chronic illness) are even more depressing (unless you live in south-west London, of course). In Richmond, women and men can anticipate a 'healthy' life of over 70 years, whereas for the women and men in the East End, there is almost 20 years' difference in the calculated span of their healthy lives (ONS 2013a).

Social inequality of health in grey and green boroughs

Table 11.2. Same town, worlds apart

London borough of Richmond (4% unemployment)	Life expectancy
Men	81.5 years (of which 70.3 considered healthy)
Women	86 years (of which 72.1 considered healthy)
London borough of Tower Hamlets (13.4% unemployment)	**Life expectancy**
Men	76.7 years (of which 55.6 considered healthy)
Women	81.9 years (of which 54.1 considered healthy)

Source: ONS 2013a, table 2.

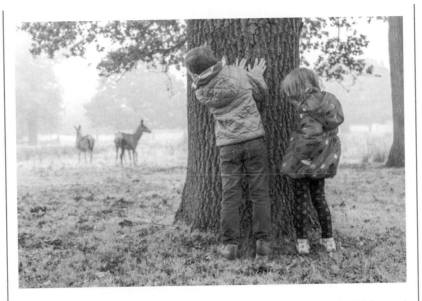

Stag party: extending over 955 hectares, the royal park in Richmond
– the largest in London – is so large that herds of fallow and red
deer roam freely. By contrast, the three largest parks in the whole of
Tower Hamlets put together only cover 120 hectares.

But how much of this sad situation is related directly to the provision (or
non-provision) of urban greenspace, and how much can be laid at the door
of social and economic status and the closely related lifestyle choices that all
too often come with the territory? A study by academics working in two
Scottish universities specifically addressed that question head on: it convinc-
ingly shows that it is indeed proximity to greenspace, rather than solely your
salary, that can significantly impact beneficially upon your health. The
research by Richard Mitchell and Frank Popham looked at a massive database selected from the records of 40,813,236 persons below retirement age
in the UK. The urban samples selected were then grouped into income
bands (which included the most deprived) and related to their proximity to
urban greenspace. These groups were then classified by various ailments
and by age at death. Significant positive associations were recorded between
all groups, regardless of income, when proximity to greenspace was measured against all causes of death and against circulatory diseases. In other
words, it seems that living close to a park has a beneficial impact on your
health regardless of your salary; conversely, the less exposure to urban
greenspace you have, the less healthy you are likely to be, again, regardless
of salary. They concluded that urban "environments which promote good
health may be the key in the fight to reduce health inequalities" (Mitchell

and Popham 2008, 1658). It was not differing access to healthcare systems or the relative distribution of wealth that seems to have made the real difference: it was the park.

Chapter 12

CENTRAL PARK

Great things are done when men and mountains meet;

This is not done by jostling in the street.

William Blake (1757–1827)

Urban greenspace: a microbiological necessity

Living in the wild, wide open was normal for our uncivilised ancestors, and we still need at least a flavour of that normality in our modern lives. Green is good, as the studies in the previous chapter show: living near a 'natural' environment is associated with long-term health benefits including a longer lifespan, reduced cardiovascular disease and fewer psychiatric problems. But why should that be so? The answer lies in what is arguably the most paradigm-shifting study discussed in this book: it is based on the remarkable research conducted by UCL microbiologist Professor Graham Rook and his colleagues. He has viewed the issue from several angles, including a consideration of the psychological effects that looking at or walking in greenspace often produces. The impact on cerebral blood flow, blood pressure and salivary cortisol can all be measured (Rook 2013), as can mood enhancement through mobile electroencephalograms (Aspinall et al. 2013).

One evolutionary explanation for this positive response to greenspace and bluespace is that it is a reminder of a fertile and welcoming habitat, the type of landscape of plenty that human hunter-gatherers were (and clearly still are) naturally drawn to (Frumkin 2001). There may well be more than a grain of truth in this, but it's an argument that's hard to prove. More importantly, there seems to be no direct connection between the measurable, agreeable but transient and short-term psychological uplift gained by walking through a park (at least in broad daylight), and how that might be translated into long-term health benefits.

Alternatively, might the proximity to urban greenspace be more conducive to regular exercise, and, if so, might it be the physical activity that benefits wellbeing, rather than the park itself? After all, you could exercise regularly indoors in the gym, rather than in the great outdoors on a dark December morning. Studies such as those reported on by Barton and Pretty (2010) argue that mood and self-esteem show marked improvement after exercise in a park or other greenspace, irrespective of duration, intensity, location, gender, age or health status. This is an encouraging result for those on the park side of the debate: green exercise provides an immediate and demonstrable positive effect in the short term. But how deep or genuinely long-lasting such mental benefits are remains unclear. This is an important question for the designers of the next generation of high-density cities, since there will be little space to spare. If they are to provide a healthy environment for the inhabitants, should the new towns of tomorrow have more indoor gyms, should they have larger parks, and what proportion of the two would be most cost-effective in delivering urban wellbeing?

Away in a manger

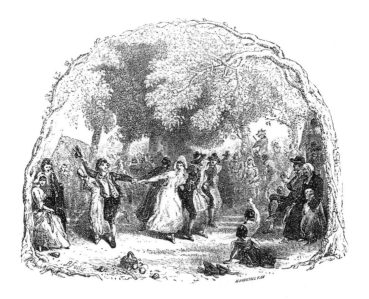

Figure 12.1. Urban greenspace: essential, and not just for social and health benefits.

Professor Rook provides an answer and an explanation that goes rather deeper than landscape appreciation – for whatever reason – while focusing on a key component of our wellbeing. In addition to close consideration of our nutritional and activity regimes, continuing good health also requires an effective immune system. But can the process of urbanisation itself be detrimental to our body's ability to fight infection and disease? As long ago as 1820, the causes and possible treatments for hay fever were being discussed by Dr John Rostock. It was observed that farmers (but more significantly their children) never suffered from this ailment: indeed, it was seen as an aristocratic affliction: "there can be no doubt that, if not wholly confined to the upper classes of society, it is rarely, if ever, met with but among the edu-cated" (Blackley 1873, 7). In an attempt to explain this social situation, it was initially suggested that it was the actual working of the trained mind that made one more prone to catarrhus aestivus (Blackley 1873, 161–162). Although this could be classified as an early example of the social determi-nants of health, its roots ran rather deeper, as Professor Rook has shown (Rook 2012). The cause lay not so much in the income of the sufferers, but in the clean, closeted upbringing of their offspring in their earliest, most formative weeks – far removed from any farmyard. Epidemiological research has now shown that children exposed to farms and farming environments have increased protection against the development of asthma and allergies in childhood when compared to those living in less rural environments (see e.g. von Mutius and Vercelli 2010).

It is from direct contact with plants and animals that we derive the macro-organisms, micro-organisms and microbiota that live and thrive on our skin and in the gut. We are not born with these microbiota: they are all derived from the external environment after birth, from the soil, from plants and animals, from the air or from contact with other humans. For millions of years they have been invading and inhabiting humans and their predecessors and, crucially, have co-evolved roles in the regulation of the human immune system. Some were benign, others were potentially harmful, but they needed to be tolerated if the benefits were to be experienced. These tiny organisms work together to provide us with our own individual ecosystem service: without them, our susceptibility to allergies, autoimmunity and inflammatory bowel disease is much increased. The same situation has been observed in other creatures as well as humans, as recent UK studies of piglets have shown. In one experiment, siblings from the same litters were divided into two groups, some staying on the farm, while the others were reared in hygienic isolator-units. It was shown that, in contrast to those from the isolators, for those reared on the farm there was a profound and positive development of the regulatory components of the mucosal immune system and to immune responses to food proteins (Lewis et al. 2012). There are, it seems, considerable long-term health benefits for those born in mangers.

Talking of births, the pros and cons of caesarean section (C-section) delivery are often in the news, but it seems that consideration of our evolutionary microbiota has added fuel to this debate. The nutritional epidemiologist Changzheng Yuan and her team at the Harvard School of Public Health looked at the records of 22,068 people, of whom 22% were born by C-section (Yuan et al. 2016). It seems that those delivered by this method were 30% more likely to be at risk of obesity as children (between 9 and 12 years old). Even more telling was the statistic that of the 12,903 people with brothers and sisters, those delivered by C-section were 64% more likely to grow up obese than their own siblings, given that they had been delivered vaginally. This strongly suggests that the range of micro-organisms in the mother's birth canal – for example, more bifidobacteria and fewer staphylo-cocci – seem to provide a major long-term health benefit for the baby should it pass through that canal and absorb the microbiota en route. This is a truly extraordinary evolutionary determinant of our health and a strong argument for 'natural births', provided, of course, there are no other more complicated health issues to contend with.

And the story does not end there. An extended period of breastfeeding was known to reduce the frequency of infections in children and to reduce the risk of them becoming overweight, although the underlying mechanism was unclear. But now a study conducted in 2015 on a group of 225 children in northern Finland suggests that the long-term metabolic benefits of breast-feeding are conveyed by the intestinal maternal microbiota (Korpela et al. 2016). However, the study also suggests that the use of antibiotics with those children seems to weaken the positive effects of extended breastfeeding.

Immunology and co-evolution

To paraphrase the introduction to one of Graham Rook's important reports (Rook et al. 2014): our immune system gradually evolved with us during the millennia we lived as hunter-gatherers. It required input from at least three sources which are sometimes referred to collectively as the 'old friends'. First there were the commensal microbiota, transmitted to us by our mothers and other family members; then there were organisms from the natural environ-ment that modulate and diversify those commensal microbiota; and finally there were the old infections that could persist relatively harmlessly in small, isolated hunter-gatherer groups. Our bodies learned to tolerate such organ-isms, and they co-evolved roles with us in the development and regulation of our immune systems.

By contrast, 'crowd infections', such as childhood virus infections, evolved later when the development of intensive agriculture and animal husbandry supported much larger communities, leading to urbanisation. Unlike the old friends, these crowd infections did not evolve immunoregulatory roles, sim-ply because the host was either killed or obtained complete immunity, and thus the infections could not live on or develop in discrete hunter-gatherer populations. Although modern western lifestyles, and the associated medical practices, all but eradicated many of the 'old' infections, immunoregulatory disorders have noticeably increased. In today's more clinical world, our immune system's input has become far more dependent upon microbiota and the natural environment. However, living in towns decreases our expo-sure to that natural environment, while simultaneously increasing our exposure to the crowd infections that lack immunoregulatory roles (Rook et al. 2014).

Thus, for those born in towns in high-income countries, it seems that many will face increases in chronic inflammatory disorders, caused partly by the failure of the immune system to respond appropriately. This seems to be because an urban child's immune system, having had only minimal exposure to microbiota, will not have 'learned' to recognise or differentiate between beneficent strains or harmful pathogens. The poorly educated immune system consequently makes inappropriate responses to what it wrongly thinks are attacks on the body, which can lead to autoimmune diseases such as multiple sclerosis. Such incorrectly identified attacks on otherwise harmless allergens can trigger allergic disorders such as hay fever, for example, while those in the gut can precipitate ulcerative colitis or Crohn's disease (Rook 2013, 18363).

This research provides a major reason why towns (or, more correctly, reduced engagement with nature in an urban environment) could be bad for our physical health: we still need the micro-organisms that only animals, plants, trees and soil can give us. Growing up in a city that has concreted over the good earth and filled its buildings with conditioned air will not support your immune system. On the other hand, living close to urban greenspace, gardening, walking outdoors and growing up with pets could ensure that you absorb sufficient microbiota to support a robust immune system. Graham Rook makes particular mention of pets, noting that "the microbiota in dust from households with dogs is significantly richer and more diverse than that found in homes without pets", or at least without pets that do not venture outdoors. He goes on to comment that the exposure of humans, especially children, to animals such as dogs "seems to provide some protection against allergic sensitization and allergic disorders" (Rook 2013, 18364). He argues that humans have co-evolved with canine microbiota ever since the domestication of the dog, and possibly even earlier than that.

Man's best friend

The taming and domestication of the grey wolf (*Canis lupus*) seems to have begun tens of thousands of years ago. DNA studies suggest that dogs began separating from the wolf lineage some 100,000 years ago, but there are fossils of wolf bones in association with early humans even earlier than that (Derr 2011). Studies show that orphaned wolf pups taken before they are 21 days old can be reared and easily tamed by humans – a neat reversal of the Romulus and Remus saga. It may also well be that some scavenging wolves were happy to live a semi-feral life close to human hunting camps: they would benefit from left-over meat and bones and, in return, serve as guard dogs or even hunting dogs without any significant genetic change. The urban fox, now so familiar in London, Bristol and many other cities, could stand as an example of the first stage in such a symbiotic process. In 2008, examination of material excavated in the late 19th century from Goyet Cave in Belgium identified a 31,700-year-old dog (*Canis lupus familiaris*), a large and powerful animal which ate reindeer, musk oxen and horses (Germonpré et al. 2009).

With the gradual adoption of animal husbandry in the Neolithic era, however, unreconstructed wolves or powerful hunting dogs might have become less useful. It may have been at this stage that different types of more domesticated dogs may have been specifically bred, such as the collie used for herding (rather than hunting) sheep and cattle. These new breeds would then have been required to keep wolf packs at bay to protect the herds and flocks. Thus it seems that man has been living with wolves and dogs (and therefore their associated rich diversity of microbiota) for far longer than he has been living in towns.

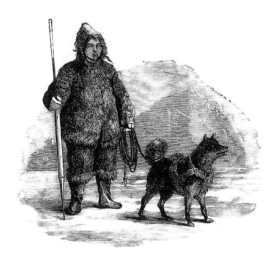

Figure 12.2. Man's best friend: arguably the first wild animal 'domesticated' by humans.

Microbiota and psychological stress

Professor Rook's crucial work goes even further than considering various physical ailments, because he has shown that if our urban bodies cope ineffectively with inflammation, then there can also be negative psychiatric consequences. This is because the same organisms and processes that help our immune system to combat inflammations also modulate brain development, cognition and mood. Consequently, if our immune system is working at a reduced level while we are suffering from psychosocial stress, the effects are exaggerated. This crucial link between psychiatric disorders and chronic inflammatory disorders – another evolutionary determinant of health – requires further detailed research by immunologists, epidemiologists, neuroscientists and psychiatrists. A possible solution suggested by the Eden Protocol may lie in the extended greening of conurbations, the keeping of pets and universal, regular access to gardens, allotments and parks. In such ways, nature might improve our immune systems for us, given that we start early enough.

There are other vital uses for micro-organisms in the soil: they are likely to be the source of the next generation of antibiotics that will be used by the medical profession to treat or contain infection. Since the 1940s, antibiotics such as penicillin and streptomycin transformed medicine, providing effective cures for most infections. However, resistance to those compounds has accelerated with their increasingly widespread use and overuse, and it has not proved possible to produce synthetic antibiotics of a suitable strength to replace or supersede them. Professor Kim Lewis and his team at Northeastern College of Science in Boston, Massachusetts are experimenting by literally growing robust uncultured organisms in the soil from which a 'new' antibiotic, termed teixobactin, is being developed (Ling et al. 2015). Clearly, the living soil is a key player in keeping us mentally and physically healthy, and for helping us to fight infection: our cities should therefore have as much earth exposed as is practical.

Which just leaves us with the next set of questions for tomorrow's town planner. First, which particular plants, shrubs and trees should be planted in (or be allowed to colonise) our towns in order to attract the better class of micro-organism that would provide the maximum health benefits? Then we need to ask how many trees per head of population there should be: is one oak better for us than six birches? Graham Rook suggests that, if urban populations are indeed obliged to look to the natural environment "to provide an appropriate airborne microbiota, then multiple small, widely distributed urban greenspaces of high microbial quality might suffice as supplements to a core of larger recreational parks" (Rook 2013, 18367). He goes on to comment on the vogue for roof gardens, vertical gardens on urban walls and urban greenspaces specifically designed to promote habitats for birds, bees and insects, or those laid out to capture rainwater to prevent the overwhelming of drainage systems during storm events. An unintended but highly welcome secondary function of all such sites would be to increase the population and availability of urban microbiota. So, even if there is little room for laying out a new large park, the streets and even the houses themselves can be (and should be) greened with trees, window boxes or flowerbeds.

Greening the city: biophilia, biodiversity and positive interaction

Having presented evidence supporting the case for urban wellbeing in a greened city, the next stage is to consider some of the topographical practicalities of a more 'natural' city environment. Today, there are a number of different types of urban greenspace (and, of course, bluespace) that city populations do (or could) have access to. The range is extensive, and clearly reflects the artificiality of the division between 'town' and 'country', between 'natural' and 'artificial', between 'greenspace' and 'greened space'. In spite of much building in concrete, brick and glass, the number of trees, gardens, parks and open spaces in many English towns is significant, and seems to be increasing. The following discussion considers urban greenspace from the perspective of human evolution, looking at the very closely interlinked issues of engagement with nature (or biophilia), the need for physical activity and for social interaction, and last, but by no means least, the promotion of biodiversity (including those life-saving microbiota).

Urban greenspace, greened space and physical activity

In the fight against obesity and its associated evils, the importance of regular exercise cannot be overstressed. For those with sedentary occupations, for example, the opportunity to walk, run or cycle through a park or through quiet, attractive greened streets will have profound health benefits. Taking such exercise as a leisure activity is fine, but incorporating such a regime – partially or fully – into your everyday commute is an even better option. However, this obviously depends on the time available, where you live and where you work, and how greened and relatively traffic-free the neighbouring streets are. It is accepted that busy towns cannot be entirely given over to open parkland, but at least some of the street network can be greened, pedestrianised or traffic-calmed. The more pleasant the urban streetscape, the more conducive the environment will be to promoting human locomotion as the norm. Crucially, approaches to schools should be designed with this in mind, for if children learn the habit of walking to school every day, then the long-term benefits of acquiring such a daily behaviour are very considerable.

Participation in many sports provides both physical and social activity, but also needs support from the urban planner in the form of playing fields and pitches. Although some of the most memorable matches are played with jumpers for goalposts (with a winning score of 10–9), facilities such as changing rooms and staff are required to foster and encourage the longer term development of the sporting habit. Over and above whatever personal health benefits might ensue (as Chapter 9 showed), there are very significant societal advantages to widening access to regular, organised sporting regimes.

In addition to formal football pitches, there are also other ways of playing outdoors. Wild Zones are described as a 'new' form of public space, offering opportunities to interact directly with the environment, and thus differ from formal gardens, parks or playing fields (www.wild-zone.net). They are designated places dedicated to adventure, creativity and play in nature, where adults and children can have fun with mud and water, or create sculptures from natural materials, or houses, dens and shelters from branches, leaves and rocks. They are usually areas at the edges of larger parks or nature reserves, or might be established over time on post-industrial brownfield sites. For modern urban children, these zones can offer a brief window into a pre-urban semi-Palaeolithic world, designed to address what has been described as the 'nature-deficit disorder'. The (temporary) rewilding of children is a concept that would resonate with the young Heathcliff and Cathy, and also with the generation that grew up alongside London's overgrown bombsites before health and safety was invented.

Working with nature: participatory urban greenspace

Key tenets of the protocols associated with the evolutionary determinants of health include engagement with nature (which includes accruing the microbiota essential for our immune system), physical activity (particularly in the open air), delivering stimulating and challenging opportunities and fostering a sense of community by providing a neighbourhood focus. All of these issues are neatly addressed by city farms, of which there are now 15 operating in the Greater London area, for example. One of the key issues underpinning this remarkable recent expansion is that the initial impetus for a particular project has often been provided by a determined community group, rather than a local authority fulfilling a statutory obligation. As a consequence, there have sometimes been serious issues regarding the longevity and sustainability of such schemes. That said, the tangible and intangible benefits provided by city farms have been ably demonstrated, making a sound case for the continued maintenance and indeed expansion of such schemes.

The first of the current generation of London's city farms was established in Kentish Town, Camden some 40 years ago. The distribution of these farms today is highly significant, since the greatest concentration by far lies in the aggressively urban inner-city boroughs. Camden, Islington, Hackney, Newham, Southwark and Lambeth all now have one farm each, with Tower Hamlets supporting no less than three. In this central core, only two boroughs do not, as yet, have a city farm of their own: Lewisham, which certainly deserves one, and the eponymous City itself – the financial district managed by the Corporation of London. Even though 'city' is used to describe the farms, this borough is simply too small and crowded to swing a cat, let alone milk a cow. The communities in the 19 rather greener outer boroughs seem to have felt less need to nurture such initiatives, there being but six such city farms between them.

These schemes are regularly visited by families for a stimulating, often unpredictable, day out, and serve as attractive and valuable open-air class-rooms for local schoolchildren living far from the open countryside. The majority of the city farms also show the socially beneficial impact that phys-ically working with animals and plants provides. Most farms provide positive work-experience placements, and many run courses that accommodate those with autism or with learning or behavioural problems, the homeless, young offenders and the unemployed. These services are provided under the umbrella of the Care Farming concept (see e.g. Hassink and van Dijk 2006). This has a long tradition in, for example, the Netherlands, Norway, the United States and Australia (Velde et al. 2005). It is relatively novel in the UK, but is expanding fast, with now at least 76 farms across the country (Sempik and Aldridge 2006).

The unique environment found on city farms can often touch those to whom urban society has not always been kind, allowing individuals to reorientate themselves through the telling combination of engaging with nature, hands-on physical activity and positive social interaction, as well as exposure to more diverse microbiota. Clients can be referred to the farms by social services, the prison service, youth offending teams, community drug teams, education authorities, pupil referral units and behavioural support units.

Such positive therapeutic horticultural practices need not, of course, be confined solely to city farms, since programmes can be run wherever there is suitable land, as has been done at a hospital in Wokingham (Gladwell 2007), and with whoever it might benefit: there is even documented evi-dence of the value of such work with victims of torture (Linden and Grut 2002). Reported benefits range from improved physical health, self-esteem and wellbeing; an increase in self-confidence, independence, personal responsibility and social skills; enhanced trust in other people; and the for-mation of a work habit. There is some debate as to whether it is the removal of the individual from the environment associated with the initial problems that provides the benefit, or if it is the farm itself (with its supportive work-ers, physical regime and plants): common sense would suggest that it's a positive combination of the two. And then there are the animals which are far less judgemental than humans: the Shetland pony who is a friend to all, for example; animals that give and accept affection unconditionally but need to be fed and cared for each day (Ewing et al. 2007; Hine et al. 2008).

The animal kingdom can also be glimpsed in parks that have a pets' corner or children's zoo facility. While not offering the same range of activities provided by city farms, they do provide children (and adults) with the opportunity to observe and interact with animals and birds. These can be found in many corners of London – for example, at Coram's Fields in Holborn, Battersea Park, Crystal Palace, Horniman Gardens in Forest Hill, Maryon Wilson Park in Charlton and Queen's Park in Brent. There is also a large zoo in Regent's Park, although the entrance fee is rather higher than that for the city farms. Then there are several nature reserves staffed by the London Wildlife Trust (www.wildlondon.org.uk) including Camley Street Natural Park in King's Cross, the East Reservoir Community Garden in Stoke Newington, the Centre for Wildlife Gardening in Peckham, at Sydenham Hill Wood, at Crane Park Island in Twickenham and at the Gunnersbury Triangle in Chiswick.

A new addition to the capital's menageries is London's first 'cat cafe', which opened in Bethnal Green Road, Shoreditch in 2014. This is a place where cats from various rescue centres may be stroked and communicated with by humans who are unable to keep pets in an urban flat. The concept originated in Taiwan in 1998, blossomed in Tokyo and subsequently spread across Asia and into Europe. There are also records of rabbit cafes and even a goat cafe in Japan. Their continuing success seems to reflect a clear need within high-density urban populations for direct contact with the animal world. Biophilia is a deep human need, as the popularity of wildlife programmes in our TV schedules shows, but this chapter has demonstrated that there are myriad ways in which even inner-city dwellers can engage far more directly with our fellow creatures.

Fruits of the earth

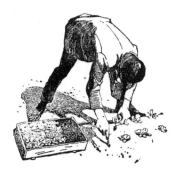

Figure 12.3. Participatory urban greenspace: working with nature.

The enhanced value of houses with gardens is well known to estate agents and also to those residents who devote time and energy to them (see e.g. Richards 2005). But for the many citizens without private gardens, their own participatory urban greenspace, other solutions have been developed. The beginnings of the allotment movement in the UK can be traced back to the late 18th century, with the renting out to local labourers of farmland and other strips (allotments) upon which a variety of crops might be grown. This practice expanded as English cities industrialised: the trade unions welcomed an initiative that enabled their workers to feed themselves cheaply (especially during periods of escalating unemployment), while employers saw the scheme as helping to keep their workforce out of the alehouse. However, in London the development was slow, since spare land was scarce and valuable, and there was already a vigorous tradition of professional market gardening ringing the City. By contrast, in New York and Philadelphia in the 1880s and 1890s, urban wasteland was being turned over to local people to grow food, leading to the founding of the Vacant Land Cultivation Society by Joseph Fels in 1907: idle land put to good use by idle hands. On this side of the Atlantic, in London, progress was very slow, and by 1914 there were only 140 plots allocated. All this changed with the food shortages brought about by the First World War. By 1916 there were 50 acres under cultivation by 800 plot-holders of the London Society, but this figure eventually increased following the passing of the Cultivation of Lands order that same year. The lead in obtaining land was often taken by local boroughs, rather than the London County Council, but by the end of the Great War, the allotment movement had made its mark and proved its worth. In May 1929, the first issue of the *National Allotments Journal* was published in London. By this date local authorities were allowed to obtain land for allotments by agreement, by hire or by compulsory purchase.

However, the competing pressure on urban space in London meant that, for example, 3,000 allotment-holders in Willesden lost their plots to the need for more housing. During the Second World War, with food rationed, allotments made a dramatic comeback, playing a leading role in the Dig for Victory campaign, with over a million plots nationwide. The UK figure fell as rationing ended, and by 2004 was down to some 250,000, as reported by Michael Wale to the Greater London Allotment Forum (Wale 2004). The importance of gardens and allotments in the production of food is now being more widely appreciated: it's not just a cost-saving measure, it's about quality of product and quality of life. London's allotment sites are spread across 30 boroughs, with only the Corporation of London, Kensington and Chelsea, and Westminster having none. According to the Greater London Authority website (www.london.gov.uk), the benefits of having a plot on an allotment include: a cheap source of fresh fruit and vegetables, and therefore a healthy diet; less contact with pesticides etc. if the produce is grown organically; and an excellent form of exercise in the fresh air. It is also an educational, challenging and rewarding experience that can reduce stress (snail infestation permitting), and which offers an opportunity to meet like-minded people and increases your sense of wellbeing. It is, in short, an activity that meets many of the key points in the personal health behaviour guidelines (see Chapter 15) related to the evolutionary determinants of health.

It is therefore worrying to note that, in the decade from 1996 to 2006, the number of allotments in London decreased on three levels. First, the number of sites diminished from 769 to 737, while the number of actual plots shrank from 22,319 to 20,786, a reduction in percentage terms of nearly 7%. This represents a total loss of over 87 acres of allotment land which, according to Peter Hulme's report, was equivalent to 54 football pitches (London Assembly Environment Committee 2006); alas, it was not sport that inherited most of that valuable land. It seems that, in some London boroughs, there was a 40-year waiting list for an allotment. The pendulum may have started to swing back again, however: according to a family food survey compiled by the Department for Environment, Food and Rural Affairs in 2012, the percentage of fruit and vegetables grown by households nationally has increased significantly from under 3% in 2008 to 5% in 2011. And more people are now keeping chickens, with the production of home-reared eggs doubling from 3% to nearly 6% in the same period (DEFRA 2012).

Although the golden age of the allotment may be over, many Londoners may still have the opportunity to grow at least some of their own food. A traditional allotment could be 250 square metres (approximately 300 square yards): this is a generous plot size for an individual food producer in a densely packed city like London. Perhaps a better use of space can be found in the development of community gardens and community gardening. This is a housing estate-based movement that utilises smaller plots of land, and is maintained – in theory at least – by a group of local residents acting cooperatively, rather than by individuals. To take an example, the Big Lottery funded the three-year Vacant Lot project, enabling it to set up some 20 community food-growing spaces on housing estates in the inner-city London boroughs of Camden, Hackney and Islington. The story of the Sandford Court estate in Hackney is typical (see https://vimeo.com/94638779). A resident, 83-year-old Irene Lewington, asked the environmental regeneration charity Groundwork London for help in transforming a bare concrete area into a community garden with 40 raised beds. The East London Business Alliance organised a team of corporate volunteers to help with the clearance, construction and development of the garden, together with workers from the City companies Aviva and Linklaters, and from the Home Office. The compost was provided for free by London Waste and was delivered from the EcoPark in Edmonton. Once completed, the resident plot-holders went straight to work on this new productive market garden.

It is to be hoped that such intensely urban initiatives would have met with the approval of the late John Seymour, who wrote the classic *The Complete Book of Self-Sufficiency* in 1976. He had previously worked in Africa, where he met with bushmen and learned something of the hunter-gatherer lifestyle (and, incidentally, was later posted to Abyssinia with my father, in the King's African Rifles). He may not have regarded the London planters as a fully self-sufficient unit; nevertheless, such initiatives provide not only fresh fruit and vegetables, but also exercise in the open air, social interaction and, hopefully, a more diverse collection of microbiota.

Greened city

An essential attribute of the evolutionary-concordant towns of the future should be their greenery: not just parks but greened streets lined with trees or window boxes, community gardens, city farms and traffic-free pedestrian routes as well as houses and offices with indoor plants. The resulting psychological uplift and potential for improved health, wellbeing and more effective immune systems would more than compensate for the costs involved. Indeed, much of the evidence-based research that underpinned the nature and wellbeing bill proposed in 2014 also supported the contention that our Palaeolithic genome still demands close engagement with the natural world, and most particularly in an urban environment. Rather than a garden city based on Sir Ebenezer Howard's generously sprawling designs, perhaps a greened city represents a more practical compromise between the need for high-density living and an evolutionary-concordant urban environment.

Chapter 13

OLD TOWN

The greatest and most admirable form of wisdom is that needed to plan and beautify cities and human communities.

Socrates (469–399 BC)

Unnatural habitat

In the bad old days, zoos were little more than penal colonies for captured animals: creatures were wrenched from their natural habitat to be closely caged in faraway places. Unsurprisingly they showed signs of severe psychological disturbance and physiological problems, rarely breeding successfully in such alien worlds. Indeed, 45% of primates living in captivity were likely to suffer from heart disease compared to just 4% of their contemporaries who still lived in the wild, according to Hayley Murphy of Zoo Atlanta (see https://greatapeheartproject.org).

Today, the wellbeing of animals in our zoos and wildlife parks is better understood and better catered for, with at least an attempt to mimic elements of their lost environment. The better the surroundings simulated their 'natural' habitat, the healthier the creatures were. Given that we humans are also primates, might there be a lesson for us here too? After all, some 3.4 billion people (50% of the world's population) are already urbanised, living in our own concrete zoos. But towns are not our natural habitat: for the majority of the last few million years, we and our immediate ancestors survived as hunter-gathers, living off the land in small tribal societies, working closely with nature.

What role should an enhanced understanding of our Palaeolithic genome have in modern urban design? Should new technologies and innovative engineering be the sole driving forces of our urban futures, or might research into the evolutionary determinants of health and human biology have as great a role to play? This book is not just about identifying how key elements of our hunter-gatherer past manifest themselves in 21st-century living, but how that knowledge can be applied today. In this chapter we consider how we might reconfigure our cities, townscapes and buildings on lines better suited to the physiology and psychology of the hunter-gatherer. As a consequence, our urban wellbeing would be quantifiably improved, and the cost to the National Health Service diminished. As in a modern zoo, the better our urban surroundings simulate our 'natural' habitat, the healthier we urban creatures will be.

This chapter will consider this approach in a historical context, looking at previous town planning experiments, with London used as an example of wider trends relating to urban wellbeing. But there are also a number of more recent philosophies and movements that arguably have at least some affinities to the evolutionary determinants of urban design. These include Sir Ebenezer Howard's garden cities, the Healthy Cities movement which originated in Toronto in 1984 and New Urbanism which developed in the 1970s. There are some other 'urbanisms' that, superficially at least, should be of relevance. One is Landscape Urbanism, seen by some as an approach to the reorganisation of post-industrial cities in decline, by others as a means to integrate housing, urban infrastructure and greenspace on large scales, and by others as the development of multi-phase, multi-use urban parks. It seems to be closely related to Ecological Urbanism, itself a mutation of the more ideologically driven Green Urbanism and Sustainable Urbanism schools. Architect Miguel Ruano defined it as "the development of multi-dimensional sustainable human communities within harmonious and balanced built environments" in his book *Eco-Urbanism*, published in 1998. Unsurprisingly, the broadly based concept of the evolutionary determinants of town planning, centipede-like, has feet in many camps.

Urban evolution

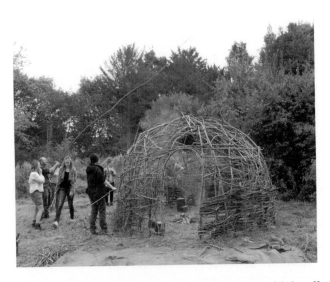

Figure 13.1. Country house: building with locally sourced
woodland materials – UCL Institute of Archaeology Field School.

The concept of the town we live with today is one that has changed over many centuries; not only have the forms, functions and types of buildings within them altered, but so too has the thinking that underpins their planning, design and subsequent development. For some civic authorities, defence may have been the prime mover, for others commerce, while, over time, interest in public health and urban wellbeing have waxed and waned. Some of these trends will be summarised later in this chapter to provide the deep context that our discussion of the evolutionary determinants of town planning demands.

Cities have not always been as impersonal, divided and dysfunctional as some seem today. One of the key questions is that of scale, since the challenges faced by a town of 250,000 souls are arguably easier to resolve than those of a city of five million or more. It is instructive to review how towns have developed historically and to identify elements in earlier plan forms from which positive and negative lessons might be learned.

Urbanism has a long history in some parts of the world. In Turkey, for example, excavations have shown that the large Neolithic settlement of Çatalhöyük dates back to the period 7500–5700 BC. The origins of Uruk, in the fertile valley of the Euphrates river in Iraq, have been traced back to 5000 BC, but it reached its largest extent in c.3000 BC, when its population probably exceeded 50,000 people. A similar size has been suggested for the city of Mohenjo Daro in Pakistan, from about 2600 BC, while the Mediterranean city-states of Ancient Greece developed rather later, in the first millennium BC.

In some parts of the world, humans have therefore been trying to adapt to urban living for almost 10,000 years. Towns which have been continuously occupied in Britain have a rather shorter history, since none can claim to be more than 1,500 years old. Nevertheless, our urban settlements have witnessed major changes in form, function and fabric over this period, but has this always represented positive progress? For how much longer can they be termed socially, economically and psychologically fit for purpose? What are the significant elements in the plan form that represent a fit, healthy settlement, and, conversely, which episodes or elements can we, with the clarity of hindsight, identify as evolutionary dead-ends or unwanted mutations in these developing town plans? At what stage could a town be said to be too large – that is, an ineffective, obese, unhealthy settlement, at least for a substantial proportion of its citizens? Learning from these history lessons, it should be possible to suggest an evolutionary-concordant approach not just to the planning of new towns in the future, but also to the reconfiguration of our current contemporary cities, where such change could prove beneficial.

Healthfulness, the first requisite

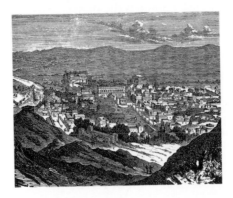

Figure 13.2. Planned town: Rome as it once was.

Writing in the first century BC, the Roman architect Marcus Vitruvius Pollio appreciated that towns were not just a random collection of streets and buildings, but that the situation, layout and location of the settlement were all important, since "healthfulness is the first requisite" of any city (Morgan 1960 [1914], 20). When choosing the location of a new town, the livers of local cattle would be examined to establish if they were firm, demonstrating that the local water was good and the pasture rich. If, however, the innards of the slaughtered cattle were diseased, then a new site would be sought. A water supply that was of little benefit to ruminants would be of no use to humans (Morgan 1960 [1914], 20). A fortified town should be set upon high ground, neither misty nor frosty, in a temperate climate and "without marshes in the neighbourhood" (Morgan 1960 [1914], 17). The streets and alleys should be laid out with due deference to the prevailing winds, since "cold winds are disagreeable, hot winds enervating, moist winds unhealthy": buildings should therefore be so constructed that just their corners face into the winds to break their force (Morgan 1960 [1914], 24–27). Taking this and other similar factors into account, it seems that a number of the evolutionary determinants of health were taken seriously, if only subconsciously, by that classical architect.

Anglo-Saxon new town

In early medieval England, the collapse of the earlier Roman administration saw the decline and fall of the first generation of British towns. The invading 'barbarian' Anglo-Saxons aggressively introduced a new language, new religions, a new tribal military culture and new economic and taxation systems to the island. By the seventh century, the warlike Saxons had also begun developing a new concept of towns – settlements that owed little (if anything) to the urbanised classical world. They initially operated as undefended trading centres for the independent tribal regions, and were known as 'wics', such as Ipswich (Suffolk), Hamwic (Southampton, Hampshire), Fordwic (Fordwich, Kent), Jorvik (York) and Lundenwic (Aldwych, London).

In the ninth century, England suffered further attacks and invasions by Danish marauders on an alarming scale, and this was the catalyst for the next major development in urbanisation, with a new generation of defended towns founded to provide better security for the beleaguered English. The 'Burghal Hidage', a list of the names, locations and comparative sizes of these urban centres, survives from the period (Hill 1969, 84–92). The text has been studied in detail, while archaeologists have investigated many of these new towns (e.g. Baker and Brookes 2013), so consequently we now have a much clearer picture of Anglo-Saxon town life. Such settlements were developed during the time of King Alfred the Great, the legendary King of Wessex. This was a man who believed that towns should integrate three cardinal elements – defensive, economic and religious – and thus accommodate men who fight, men who work and men who pray. Although much overlain by successive changes in function and building types, the success of this particular Saxon settlement type can be gauged by its stubborn (if admittedly fragmentary) topographical survival beneath many of our major English towns today.

The topography of tenth-century London, for example, is of considerable interest to the discussion of the evolutionary determinants of town planning. The settlement made use of the ancient masonry walls that had been built in the early third century to defend Roman Londinium. The initial compact settlement core for the craftsmen and traders was just under 1 km in length and about 350 metres in width, and thus occupied only a quarter of the defendable intramural area (Milne 1990). Between the western edge of that settlement core and the west gate leading out of the City was the precinct of the mother church of St Paul's; to the north (beyond Cheapside) and east (beyond Billingsgate) of the settled area there were substantial tracts of urban greenspace – fields within the walls. These were variously utilised, as the occasion demanded, for pasturing livestock overnight, as cattle markets, as market gardens and, in times of crisis, as temporary mustering sites for the regional militia or to accommodate refugees from the surrounding countryside (Milne 2002, 120–127). Immediately outside the walled area were the field systems farmed by the citizens themselves, and thus London had already established its own essential food-producing 'green belt' 1,000 years before Sir Ebenezer Howard published his concept of the garden city. For the Anglo-Saxons, urban greenspace was far more than mere landscaping: it was essential to the functioning of the town and for the lives and livelihoods of its inhabitants.

Great rebuilding

Without clear, centralised town planning policies and guidelines in place, even towns that were initially laid out with the clearest of visions have a habit of accruing unanticipated accretions to accommodate population levels that cannot be absorbed easily. Although it is possible to impose a brand new plan directly over an ageing, extant town, as Baron Haussmann's new Paris shows, the problems and costs are far more complex than laying out a new town on a new site. Often the opportunity to rebuild an old town that has outgrown its initial plan form only comes in the wake of a major disaster, such as Constitución after the earthquake and tsunami hit Chile in 2010, or Tokyo after the fire-bombing in the Second World War. Fire was indeed the scourge of many towns from antiquity to the present age. This is certainly the case with London, a city that has suffered many such conflagrations, and consequently many such rebuildings. Two infamous traumas are the Great Fire of 1666 and the Blitz of the 1940s, both of which saw a new town arise from the ashes of the old. Much can be learned from comparing the town planning response in the late 17th century to its previous incarnation: the features which were retained are as interesting as those which were summarily discarded, highlighting the elements that were considered obsolete or obstructive. In 1667–1670, the street plan was largely retained, but the streets themselves were widened; the broad patterns of neighbourhood layout, property ownership and parish structure were retained, although over 30 of the smaller parishes were subsumed by larger neighbouring churches; strict uniform building regulations were imposed across the board, with the blanket banning of timber-framed housing.

Surprisingly, the plan for the new London has been seen by some as a wasted opportunity, since the impractical but ambitious plans initially proposed by architects such as Sir Christopher Wren were not implemented (CoL 1944, 11). Indeed, no less a figure than Nikolaus Pevsner dismissed the adopted plan as "narrow, confused and medieval … hardly anything was done" (Pevsner 1973, 63). But anyone who has read T. F. Reddaway's detailed account of what was actually achieved from 1667 to 1711 is forced to take a contrary view. His book, published in 1940, just as the city he described was being destroyed by fire yet again, shows that the rebuilding of London after the Great Fire was a triumph (it would have certainly met with the approval of the New Urbanists).

The regeneration works were carried out with speed, for within ten years much of the town was up and running, and work on the new churches and public buildings had also begun in earnest. An elegant facade of red brick terraces and white Portland stone churches had replaced the cramped and overcrowded medieval plan. The churches, with their idiosyncratic towers and steeples sailing above the uniform roof lines, provided attractive foci for the City's neighbourhood parishes, while the great dome of the mother church of St Paul's, once completed, dominated the skyline from whatever direction London was approached. This was thus a very modern city, modelled on architectural styles copied from a wider Europe, but still representing a culture in which the tallest buildings were churches. The final result was recorded in 1707 by John Woodward, the professor of physics at Gresham College. In a letter written to his colleague, Sir Christopher Wren, one of the six commissioners responsible for the new plan, Woodward describes the Great Rebuilding in these glowing terms:

> So many thousands of houses ... built in such a manner as to render them not only more convenient ... but even superior in design and architecture to the palaces of princes elsewhere ... Then, by means of the enlargement (widening) of the streets, and of the great plenty of good water conveyed to all parts, of the common sewers and other like contrivances, such provision is made for a free access and passage of air, for sweetness, for cleanliness, and for salubrity, that it is not only the finest, but the most healthy City in the world. (Reddaway 1940, 300)

This healthy new city introduced into English towns, on a scale hitherto not seen in this country, the now familiar streetscape of brick-built terraces opening directly on to the street. The London Rebuilding Act 1667 laid out the strict regulations governing the construction of these uniform terraces (Milne 1986, 116–119): buildings on by-streets or lanes were to be two storeyed, those fronting streets of note or overlooking the Thames were to be three storeyed, while those fronting the high and principal streets could be of "the greatest bigness" (i.e. four storeys). Not only was the City's social class structure thus expressed architecturally, but it also meant that the height of the buildings was directly proportional to the width of the streets. Consequently, all thoroughfares, however narrow, would not be overshadowed by over-large buildings, blocking out the natural light with their over-large shadows. Such a consideration was of some importance before the introduction of artificial gas or electric light.

There is a lesson here for modern town planners: in many narrow city lanes prior to the Second World War, tall office buildings frequently resorted to placing mirrors outside their windows in a desperate attempt to increase the light levels. How many city streets today only see direct sunlight at midday (if at all), as a direct consequence of the mismatch of narrow streets and buildings with far too many storeys?

A final point that is evident in the design of late 17th-century London was that the tallest buildings were still churches; today they are banks. (Discuss.) A comparison of the fate of the vestiges of the post-Great Fire City with that of the late 20th-century redevelopment after the horrors of the Blitz is also telling. Over 300 years after the London Rebuilding Act of 1667, surviving elements of that townscape are now lovingly listed, while key elements of the latter (e.g. Paternoster Square, Bucklersbury House, the Highwalk) were demolished and replaced within 50 years.

Any town laid out on the pragmatic principles shown in late 17th-century London should provide 'healthfulness' for its fortunate citizens, but alas not all settlements were initially built with such foresight. Certainly by the early 19th century, it was clear that no advice from Sir Christopher Wren had been sought, and no cattle had been slaughtered to determine whether many new English industrial towns had been built in healthy locations. The rising mortality rates in the cramped and over-crowded inner-city slums could not be ignored forever. It seemed to those like Sir Edwin Chadwick, who worried about those conditions, that it was the lack of good ventilation that was primarily to blame, initially at least (Lewis 1952; Herbert 1999, 434–437). Given that the worst afflicted areas often comprised over-subdivided houses or tall tenements with fixed windows overlooking dank, dark enclosed yards, poorly circulated, putrid air was an obvious target. This is an interesting reflection on the comments of Vitruvius made 2,000 years earlier, with his discussion of the prevailing winds, building orientation and public health (discussed above).

The initial solution was therefore to re-establish the well-paved, well-drained, wind-swept open street and banish the narrow courts and blind alleys where disease-ridden, fetid air could foster sundry diseases (Herbert 1999, 435). This more regular townscape, as pioneered in the historic City of London in the 1670s and 1680s, encouraged the easier circulation of traffic, fresh air and social intercourse. It also facilitated the practicalities of laying sewers and the provision of a piped water supply. In this way, 19th-century town planners consciously accepted that "healthfulness is the first requisite" of the streetscape: urban design, public health and civic authorities were now singing, more or less, in unison.

An interesting postscript to town planning for health in London before the Second World War concerns a visionary development of the Pioneer Health Centre in the deprived working-class area of Peckham, established by George Scott Williamson and his wife Innes Hope Pearse. The modernist building, opened in 1935, provided facilities for a range of sports and social activities that the local community could organise and access for just 1 shilling per week, and included a naturally lit indoor swimming pool. All the windows in the building could be opened to allow fresh air to circulate, while the floors were cork to encourage people to exercise in bare feet. The (improving) health of all participants was monitored annually. Ironically, the ethos of this visionary experiment did not quite fit with that of the newly established National Health Service, and the centre was closed in 1950 (Pearse and Crocker 1943; Duncan 1985).

Urban visions

Some town planning philosophies that resonate, at least in part, with the evolutionary determinants of urban design are:

Garden city

The garden city movement established by Sir Ebenezer Howard in 1898 introduced social, psychological and wider environmental issues into the concept of planning for a healthy city. Howard advocated socially well-ordered town plans that embraced public parks, open spaces and tree-lined boulevards. He separated industrial zones from residential areas, built houses with gardens front and back, and surrounded the settlement core with a green belt (Howard 1902 [1898]).

This was town planning that was family and neighbourhood friendly, and also responded to a basic human need to maintain a strong and obvious relationship with a fertile landscape. The movement bore fruit in Letchworth and Welwyn, and, with some modifications, in the spate of 'new town' developments across the UK in the aftermath of the Second World War. The concept was also adopted elsewhere, at least in part, with examples in the United States, Canada, Australia, Argentina, Israel and Bhutan, for instance. Since urban greenspace and engagement with nature are key evolutionary determinants, it is easy to see why elements of the work of the garden city movement are still relevant today.

New Urbanism

New Urbanism developed in North America in the 1970s and was formally constituted in 1993. It was a reaction to urban decline, to the emergence of a culture of automobile dependency associated with the urban sprawl that saw an increasing separation of residential zones from areas where people shopped or worked. At its core are the principles of a more traditional mixed-use neighbourhood design. Walkability is a key issue, for children attending school, and for access to shops, to the defined centre of the neighbourhood and to local playgrounds. According to its charter, the new neighbourhoods:

> should be diverse in use and population; communities should be designed for the pedestrian and transit as well as the car; cities and towns should be shaped by physically defined and universally accessible public spaces and community institutions; urban places

should be framed by architecture and landscape design that celebrate local history, climate, ecology, and building practice.
(Congress for New Urbanism n.d.)

The promotion of human locomotion, the limiting of car use, the development of the concept of a community defined by the architecture and
planned topography and the provision of public spaces and urban
greenspace are all elements that can be directly related to the evolutionary determinants of town planning.

Healthy Cities

The Healthy Cities movement developed from a conference held in
Toronto in 1984. Its own charter was launched in Ottawa in 1986, after
which a major symposium held in Lisbon, hosted by the World Health
Organization, launched the European Healthy Cities Project (Tsouros
1990; Hancock 1993). By 2003, less than 20 years after its foundation,
1,300 cities in 29 countries had signed up (Rydin et al. 2012). The movement builds on the assumption that there is an 'urban advantage' (i.e.
the economic, social and health benefits of urban life outweigh the
disadvantages endured by the rural poor) and that proactive programmes which effectively address the social inequalities of health
should be implemented. It accepts that since cities are complex systems,
delivering such positive health outcomes is dependent on many varied
interactions. Some of the charter's key features which are directly or
tangentially related to the Eden Protocol include: stable ecosystems;
provision of basic needs (water, food, shelter, safety, work) for all; clean,
safe, high quality environments including adequate and affordable
housing; a diverse, vital and innovative economy; and public participation in matters relating to life, health and wellbeing.

The implications for proactive town planning are acknowledged. It is
stressed that there is a need for an urban design that is compatible with
and enhances the listed health features and consequently delivers a
quantifiably "high positive health status and a low disease status". It is
the very features of just such a health-improving urban design that we
are concerned with in this chapter, including building standards, the
built environment and physical activity, and the important relationship
with public transportation policies (Rydin et al. 2012, 13–18).

Garden cities and garden suburbs

Straight uniform streets and endless brick terraces, however clean, provided a somewhat arid facade that was not to everyone's taste, however. Sir Ebenezer Howard's garden city movement introduced issues such as the neighbourhood and the environment into the mix, with urban greenspace in all its forms holding centre stage. Although initially concerned with new foundations, many older towns adopted some of the principles behind Howard's garden city thinking, but applied them to new peripheral suburban developments. These garden suburbs often boasted semi-detached houses on spacious plots, curving streets and tree-lined cul-de-sacs. Raymond Unwin (1863–1940), a prominent architect and town planner, was influenced by the Arts and Crafts movement, by his famous contemporary – the pioneering town planner and sociologist Patrick Geddes, and by Sir Ebenezer Howard's concepts. He undertook work in various centres in Britain, as well as in some of London's new garden suburbs, at Hampstead (1905) and at Brentham, in Ealing (1907). He also did much to improve standards of working-class housing, and played a leading role in the influential Tudor Walters Committee report published just after the Great War (and the Homes Fit for Heroes campaign) as the Housing Act 1919: this advocated standards and densities based on those suggested in the garden cities report. He thus exercised considerable influence on the form of much inter-war housing and went on to be technical adviser to the Greater London Regional Planning Committee from 1929. Urban greenspace and the attendant engagement with nature were thus familiar features on the town planners' agenda in the 20th century.

Brave new worlds

But modernists had rather different views on townscapes: garden cities were now seen as too wasteful of valuable space, providing as they did a very non-intensive use of land. Howard's initial garden city concept, introduced before the motorcar had become ubiquitous, was designed around an ideal population of 32,000 – that is, some 10,000 to 15,000 houses. This is arguably too small a figure for the scale of urbanisation required in the late 21st century and beyond. The modernists proposed that higher density housing in clean, modern, well-appointed buildings could solve both social and accommodation needs: traffic, pedestrians, workplaces and residential areas would all operate more effectively if segregated. The aftermath of the Second World War, which had seen too many horrors and too many cities brutally blitzed, provided an opportunity for town planners to experiment with some of these new social, structural and architectural ideas in the design of the post-bellum city. And so while some towns were rebuilt as replicas of what had been destroyed, others were laid out as revised versions of the garden city concept, while others adopted a rather more radical modern approach.

During the Second World War, the Blitz destroyed over 50,000 inner London homes, many offices, warehouses and factories, and left vast tracts of land vacant. The London County Council and the Corporation of London were thus presented with unique opportunities to re-plan and rebuild on a visionary scale, to try to rectify the effects of haphazard and rapid urban and industrial development over the previous two centuries. The Greater London Plan of 1944 was developed by Patrick Abercrombie (1879–1957) for London County Council, and addressed the five main inter-related issues of population growth, housing, employment and industry, recreation and transport. These were considered in depth and in detail, working with a series of concentric rings imposed over the metropolitan area and beyond: this was planning on a truly regional scale. Development within the once over-crowded area designated the 'inner urban ring' would see a restricted level of housing and industry, the 'suburban ring' a mix of housing and light industry, while the 'green belt' would have far less development, other than for parkland and recreational spaces. Satellite towns would be developed beyond the green belt to accommodate the bombed-out populations from the overcrowded core to be rehomed with a better standard of housing in gardened new towns.

The communities thus created inside and outside London would inhabit an urban architecture that supported the concept of neighbourhood. The catchment areas of all new schools would be a safe and sensible walking distance, light industry and shops would be dispersed across the area, and public transport would be organised to link each neighbourhood. In 1944 some of the innermost boroughs had 0.1 acre of greenspace per 1,000 inhabitants; Abercrombie felt the ratio should be a far more generous 4 acres per 1,000 citizens. That, at least, was the vision and the dream. This last goal, like many others, was not achieved in the initial iteration of the master plan: given the dramatic ambition coupled with the limited resources and time available, it was remarkable that such a grand scheme was even started.

Another element in the plan concerned the private car: in 1910 there were less than 150,000 cars on British roads, but by 1940 that figure had increased 20-fold in just 30 years to over three million. Congestion and traffic accidents had increased in tandem, but the road network had barely changed at all. Abercrombie therefore planned a series of arterial roads and ring roads across greater London to improve traffic circulation, on the American model. A similar solution was suggested at the same time in the ancient City of London itself, the square mile set in the heart of the conurbation: here major highways were suggested both on the northern edge of the City and to the south along the riverside (CoL 1944, 19–24). These highways were intended to divert through-traffic from the centre to the extremities, but the final solutions were subject to much modification.

In this period, and indeed for decades to come, the challenges presented by the motorcar were seen in terms of building or widening roads to mitigate congestion and improve traffic flow, rather than limiting car use and curbing pollution. The car was king and had to be accommodated. The concepts of congestion charging, walkability or increasing bicycle use were not under serious consideration. In the City, the pedestrians would be segregated from the traffic on highwalks, while the residents would be segregated from their offices in the inward-looking fortress-like Barbican complex. The new commercial premises would form serried ranks of steel-framed buildings, punctuated by a sorry series of dwarfed and redundant churches, several of which were just the towers or shells of demolished buildings, half-folly, half-memorial to an obsolete past. With hindsight things might have been done differently. That said, when faced with acres of overgrown bomb sites and the need to get back to work and embrace a new normality, progress was seen as the optimistic option. In an age of austerity and ration books, modernism understood progress rather better than hindsight.

Chapter 14

URBAN REGENERATION

We shape our buildings and afterward our buildings shape us.

Sir Winston Churchill (1874–1965)

Evolutionary-concordant approach to urban design

If a modern architectural practice invited a tribe of hunter-gatherers to discuss their designs for a town plan, what revolutionary ideas might be brought to the table? How might the tribe rework the most artificial of environments into something more natural and more normal? To the best of my knowledge, such a fertile focus group has not been consulted, but for all our futures, we must review the essential evolutionary determinants of town planning. These include the need for fresh air, fresh water and fresh food; the need to facilitate human locomotion/activity levels; the need to facilitate positive health behaviours at personal and social levels; and the need to engage with nature. Such features must be addressed at many levels: in the design of streets, domestic buildings and the public realm, in the balance of the provision and accommodation of public transportation systems and private cars, and in the policy and provision regarding urban greenspace.

That some of these elements have appeared regularly on the town planners' debating table in the preceding chapter says something for their importance; even if the evolutionary rationale for their inclusion was not fully appreciated or even understood, the need to include them seemed self-evident. And where these elements were neglected or excluded, the impact on contemporary urban wellbeing was invariably negative. The message therefore seems simple enough: if you want to design a healthy city, then plan one that best accommodates our Palaeolithic genome. For the most part, the tools are already there, waiting to be used.

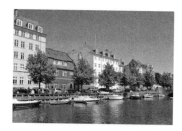

Figure 14.1. Urban greenspace, urban bluespace: summer in Copenhagen.

Evolutionary determinants of town planning

The global momentum driving the expansion of urbanisation is part and parcel of an unstoppable demographic force. We can't prevent the development of new towns or the expansion of old ones; what we can do is suggest ways to make the next generation of towns better by making them more evolutionary concordant. It is accepted that 'successful' urban settlements must have an economic rationale, be that based on heavy industry, the service industries, manufacturing, commerce, tourism or any combination of the above. But they must also provide a healthy and safe environment for their inhabitants: urban architectural design should be more than just seeing who can build the tallest tower. Issues such as human-scale social interaction, public transportation, walkability and greenspace must all be addressed if such settlements are to be considered 'healthy'. Such human-centric designs should take into account these six evolutionary determinants of town planning:

1. Fresh air

2. Fresh water

3. Fresh food (see Chapters 4 and 5)

4. Human locomotion/activity levels (see Chapters 6 and 7)

5. Evolutionary determinants of social behaviour (see Chapters 8 and 9)

6. Engagement with nature (see Chapters 11 and 12)

Those determinants all impact on town planning and urban wellbeing in many ways, negatively if they are ignored or positively if they are embraced:

1. Design of streets (1, 4, 5, 6)

2. Public transportation systems, variously defined (1, 4, 5, 6)

3. Role of private car use (in the light of 1 and 4)

4. Design of the public realm (1, 2, 4, 5, 6)

5. Residential building design and scale (1, 2, 4, 5, 6)

6. Public building and workplace design (1, 2, 3, 4, 5, 6)

7. Provision of urban green- and bluespace (1, 2, 3, 4, 5, 6)

Fresh air, fresh water, fresh food

A key feature of towns choosing to adopt the Healthy Cities Ottawa Charter of 1986 is the need to provide fresh water (so often taken for granted these days) and to address the challenges of removing wastewater and human sewage. Such systems, if badly managed or maintained, will lead to major and widespread health problems. Humans were not designed to live in such close quarters in such large numbers: disease is too easily passed on and water too easily contaminated. It has been estimated that 2.6 billion people, mainly in Asia and Africa, do not enjoy the health benefits of basic sanitation, and in 2010 a World Health Organization/UNICEF report on the subject argued that access to clean drinking water and adequate sanitation systems should be regarded as a basic human right. That such a basic evolutionary determinant of health might be written into the statute books is an interesting reflection on how far humankind has strayed from the Palaeolithic norm.

Fresh air is not something that is immediately associated with large conurbations, especially those with major industrial complexes and too many cars, or, indeed, the burning of fossil fuels. When London's homes were heated by coal fires, it was infamous for its 'pea-soupers', its foul toxic fogs. The Great Smog which blanketed the city in December 1952 was unprecedented, however, and it is claimed that it caused the death, directly or indirectly, of at least 12,000 people. It was the catalyst for the Clean Air Act 1956, which was introduced via a private member's bill rather than as a part of a manifesto commitment. This pioneering Act introduced 'smoke control areas' in cities where only smokeless fuels could be burned, starting a major movement away from solid fuels for domestic heating to a much greater reliance on electricity and gas.

Our lungs were not designed to cope with such high levels of sulphur, and neither are they able to cope with traffic fumes from diesel fuel. A report for DEFRA published in 2015 has shown that the emissions of nitrogen dioxide and the tiny diesel particulates from diesel-powered vehicles have risen steadily over the last 15 years. It goes on to suggest that 29,000 premature (i.e. avoidable and unnecessary) deaths in Britain may have been caused by such emissions. That is well over twice the number of deaths attributed to the Great Smog of 1952. Diesel fumes also raise the risk of heart attack and stroke as well as asthma attacks. Two recent studies, including one at King's College London, paint an even worse picture. One report, based on work in Tower Hamlets and Hackney, suggests that air pollution is responsible for permanently stunting the growth of children's lungs, while the other shows the damage actually starting in the womb where pregnant mothers are living in polluted areas. Toxic particles and gases emitted by diesel engines appear to be the principal culprits (see Leake 2014). However, worrying increases in the harmful pollutant called PM2.5 (such as those recorded in the London smog event between 10 and 13 March 2016) are historically linked to increases in hospital admissions and the premature death of the old and sick due to diseases of the respiratory and cardiovascular systems, according to the British Lung Foundation. Presumably another private member's bill will be required to provide the legislation needed to tackle these challenges. The fight for fresh air, a basic evolutionary determinant of health, has not yet been won on the streets of London.

As for our daily diet, that was discussed in detail in Chapters 4 and 5. All that will be mentioned here, in relation to urban food supplies, is that most of us rely on supermarkets to supply fresh fruit and vegetables. But how many of them are locally sourced? Do you make best use of your garden, if you have one, to grow at least some of your own food? Does your local authority encourage allotments or community gardening? Are there regular farmers' markets in your area? What is the quality of food served in your staff canteen, the local council offices, the school hall or the university refectory? Do your employees just have a vending machine with sugary drinks and chocolate bars in the corridor? Responsibility for what you eat is principally an individual matter, but an employer can take a responsible (or an irresponsible) approach to the health and wellbeing of their employees through the menus, facilities and social spaces provided.

Planning a city for human consumption

The next sections look at aspects of the built environment, and how the town plan itself needs to place human locomotion (rather than the car) at its heart, how it must reflect the evolutionary determinants of health and social wellbeing in its building design, and how sufficient greenspace, greened streets and greened buildings should be provided.

Garden cities or greened towns?

Just over a century after Sir Ebenezer Howard's vision first appeared in print, the Town and Country Planning Association published guidelines for local authorities on approaches to "creating garden cities and suburbs today" (Macfadyen 2013 [1938]). This document sets out ways to implement aspects of the profound, coordinated thinking on social, environmental and architectural issues that underpinned the initial garden city concept, but reworked for a 21st-century context. The cardinal principles it enshrines include a settlement that is community focused, specifically designed to be healthy and for human locomotion, but with an integrated and accessible transport system, with generous greenspace and opportunities for residents to grow some of their own food (Macfadyen 2013 [1938], 5). This encapsulates much of the evolutionary-concordant approach to town planning.

The debate really begins when the need arises to build a new town, or increase urban density or reconfigure extant townscapes in an older settlement. Creating a garden city on a blank slate is a challenge in itself, involving long timeframes, complex land purchasing and financing agreements and working within the National Planning Policy Framework and the Localism Act 2011, as well as the Housing Strategy for England, to name but a few of the hoops to be negotiated. But are the occupation densities achieved in the smaller projects practical on a larger scale? The larger and more generous the suburban layout is, the less walkable it becomes. Move forward one century, and any authority trying to house the expanding population would be thinking twice about two-storeyed properties with front and back gardens. Compromises will have to be made (e.g. smaller back gardens but larger parks) to squeeze everyone into the next generation of healthy new towns.

But if some of the more generous aspects of garden cities might have to be trimmed to fit the new world order, what of the old towns? Could they be reconfigured to become healthier? And if so, could such 'greened cities' provide models and approaches that might inform and enliven the design of tomorrow's garden cities? In many an old town, there are areas that have fallen on hard times and require renewal. The phrase used for such a process is usually 'urban regeneration', which often means little more than a few privately financed high-rise blocks of flats with retail outlets at ground level overlooking a token communal greenspace. But the term should have a deeper and more honest meaning if the redevelopments associated with it are to enjoy a long and productive life, rather than just a relatively fast financial return. Here we will consider approaches to townscapes and buildings that build on the evolutionary determinants of health and urban wellbeing.

These towns were made for walking

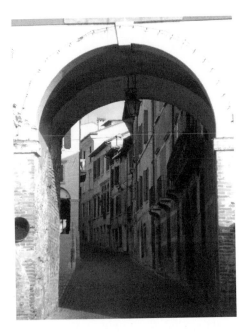

Ancient towns built by humans for humans.

'Pedestrianisation' is the term used when part, or indeed all, of a town is converted into a car-free or auto-free zone, sometimes known as a pedestrian mall. The use of delivery and emergency vehicles is allowed, but by drastically lowering the levels of car use, or by excluding them altogether, significant improvements in urban wellbeing are recorded. The air quality is improved and traffic accidents are avoided, while walking, cycling, active children's play and social interaction are all encouraged. Given so many benefits, it seems difficult to argue against such policies in modern towns.

Pedestrianisation is thought by many to be a recent phenomenon: the Lijnbaan in Rotterdam is often claimed to be the first purpose-built pedestrian street in Europe, and dates to 1953, while the first car-free shopping centre in modern England was built in Stevenage in 1959. Both were part of a brave new world, by-products of major re-planning after dreadful urban destruction during the Second World War. But many of our towns and their streets are far older than that, dating back to the centuries long before the motor car: our historic town centres were all built for pedestrians (or for horses, carts or donkeys). Rotterdam and Stevenage should not, therefore, be seen as pioneering novel concepts in urban living; they were simply returning to a tried and tested regime some hundreds or even thousands of years older. Indeed, many ancient towns (such as Lindos on Rhodes) have streets too narrow for cars, while Venice has as little need of them in this century as it had in the previous millennium.

Across Europe, it is often the historic cores of such ancient towns that are in the vanguard of new pedestrianisation, for example:

- Vienna (Austria)
- Antwerp, Brussels, Ghent (Belgium)
- Dubrovnik, Split (Croatia)
- Copenhagen (Denmark)
- Dijon, Lyon, Montpellier, Paris (France)
- Freiburg (Germany)
- Athens, Rhodes, Thessaloniki (Greece)
- Bologna, Florence, Milan, Rome, Siena, Turin (Italy)
- Krakow (Poland)
- Obidos (Portugal)
- Kremlin/Moscow (Russia)
- Malaga, Seville, Bilbao, Vitoria (Spain)
- Parts of Canterbury, Cambridge, Edinburgh, Lincoln, Oxford, York (United Kingdom)

By contrast, in North America – the land of the automobile – pedestrian malls are not as common. That said, on Mackinac Island in Michigan, the 1896 ban on horseless carriages still stands, while at least parts of New York, Boston, New Orleans and Miami Beach also share restrictions on such machines. So, will the new urban centres of the future be designed for increasing car use, or will human locomotion be at the heart of tomorrow's town planning?

Active travel, active buildings

Walking or cycling to and from school or at least for part of the route to work and back each day would be a simple solution to reducing our weight and health problems. If such a programme was adopted on a city-wide basis it would also reduce car travel, traffic congestion, air pollution, carbon dioxide and diesel emissions, noise levels and road traffic accidents.

Much of the necessary planning and design frameworks for improving urban walkability are now in place, but what makes one particular street attractive (or indeed unattractive) for pedestrians? Is it a street architecture issue, such as traffic exclusion, calming measures, tree planting or wider pavements? If local authorities are determined to make their town walkable, then a consultation exercise is required to address that question, although the answers will depend on which groups of people are asked. For active commuters heading for the centre of town, directness is often more important than scenery or townscaping, whereas for the elderly in the Netherlands, a study published in 2010 produced some interesting comments. A group of 288 people aged between 55 and 80, all living independently, were asked to comment on 25 features that related positively or negatively to the perceived attractiveness (in terms of walkability) of streets in their neighbourhood. Features that attracted unfavourable reviews included high-rise buildings or the density of dwellings, whereas positive reactions were attached to trees along the route, gardens and parks, but also bus stops, shops, catering establishments and access to the city centre. Arguably, it seems that there was an underlying purposefulness in their walking, rather than purely exercise for exercise's sake, for which circuits of the park would suffice. However, the three most critical features were litter and the tidiness of the street, its scenic value and the presence of activity or other people along the street, not all of which are the direct responsibility of the town planner. Thus aesthetics, personal security and the chance for positive social interaction also have important roles to play in the final choice of the route (Borst et al. 2008).

Putting human locomotion at the heart of a city's transport policy is most certainly evolutionary concordant. Initially it only requires a change in the wording of key documents that assume walkability is still a secondary consideration behind the needs of the private car. It can be done, as is shown by the succinct but far-reaching textual modifications suggested by Jason Gilliland's team for the Master Transport Plan for London, Ontario (Gilliland et al. 2012, 14–17), for example. But should the bill for implementing the necessary change be paid for by the transport department, the planners or the department of health? Reviews of the local transport plan take place every five years, and as more people undertake active travel, so the proportion of investment can be changed to reflect the larger number of journeys undertaken by human locomotion.

Unlike our active hunter-gatherer predecessors, many of our modern daily work patterns demand prolonged sedentary behaviours. As has been shown, these contribute to an insufficiently active lifestyle that can, in turn, be a significant predictor of cardiovascular mortality. Jobs that involve too much sitting down are bad for our health: the body was not designed for it. If the job simply can't be changed, then measures should be taken to increase physical activity rates during the journey to work, after work or back in the home.

But work patterns can (and should) be altered to make life more active, and buildings should be designed to encourage such positive health behaviour. In the drive to increase activity levels in the workplace, much attention has been given to making more use of the stairs rather than the elevator or escalator. A message prompt (in the form of a poster or other sign) reminding the viewer of the health benefits of using the stairs, rather than the lift, seems to be an effective way of encouraging stair use. These are set up at the point of choice, where the viewer has to consciously decide which route to take. But would a single sign increase use just of the stairs next to it, or would the message carry over to the next flight reached by the walker? An experiment with such signs was undertaken in a shopping mall on two different stair/escalator pairings, set some 25 m apart on either side of an atrium. Over a period of two weeks some 70,000 ascending pedestrians were monitored. On the first flight (the one with the signs) stair use increased by 161%, while on the second flight, without prompts, stair use increased by 143%. A subsequent five-week monitoring period recorded continued high stair use, even after the banners had been removed. It seems that behaviour had been changed by this relatively modest intervention (Webb and Eves 2007).

Studies of similar message-led projects have been shown to increase stair climbing by 50–129% in some situations, while the addition of banners on the stair treads themselves has proved to be even more persuasive, with increases of 127–129% recorded (Webb and Eves 2006, 49). Oliver Webb and Frank Eves also investigated the form of the message itself, comparing those that say, for example, 'free exercise' with others that emphasise the health benefits, for example, 'keeps you fit'. Those that suggest a reward or positive consequence seem to be more effective as persuaders. If such messages are accompanied by the logo from a creditable source (e.g. a government department), then they may also have more impact (Webb and Eves 2006, 53–54), but that might depend on the building and government in question. Banners thus have their uses, but might not the office receptionist be instructed to proffer directions encouraging all visitors to ignore the lift and only make use of the stairs ("up two flights, first on the right")?

Moving on, might not the very design of the building have a major part to play? First of all, if the stairwell is not well lit, clean or colourful it will not attract many climbers on its own merits; if it looks like a no-go area, that's how it will be treated, regardless of the carefully placed slogans. Indeed, in many office blocks, while the lift shaft is centrally placed, in clear sight of the front door, the stairwell is tucked away to one side, often uncarpeted, blandly decorated and largely unused save for the annual fire drill. But in a low-fat, active office building, a grand staircase occupies pride of place in the foyer, with light-filled landings replete with seating, artwork and plants. Staff simply prefer to walk up the stairs (no encouraging messages required), only using the lift when heavy loads or other requirements dictate otherwise. Good building design can make the right decisions for you, as architects such as Allies and Morrison have shown in their use of stairwells as key internal office features, for example. It's not just about offices, of course: public buildings can also be active. The redesign of the Museum of Modern Art in New York by Yoshio Taniguchi has an impressive, prominently located staircase to discourage over-use of the elevators, for example. Then there's the famous flight in the Odenplan metro station in Stockholm, Sweden. In 2009, a Volkswagen team transformed it into a set of musical piano keys: these have proved very popular with commuters, with 66% preferring them to the escalator.

Room with a view

Clearly, the built environment does affect the learning progression of our schoolchildren, but we weren't born to be inside all day. Research by the Heschong Mahone Group in California suggested that the more daylight a school captures, the more attendance increases and the more test results improve (from 5% to 14%), while learning rates could be enhanced by up to 26% (Heschong Mahone Group 1999). A school complex and an associated curriculum thoughtfully redesigned on evolutionary-concordant principles could thus improve the learning environment (Barrett et al. 2013) and impact positively on their long-term health as well.

Studies have also been done on the design of hospitals: a seminal paper published in 1984 showed that the time patients needed for recovery was reduced by up to 8.5% if they were in rooms with windows affording a suitably therapeutic green view. The research was conducted in Pennsylvania, and involved study of the records of patients who were recuperating from a standard cholecystectomy operation between 1972 and 1981. They were laid up in two sets of rooms which were identical in all respects, apart from the view from the single window: in one wing the view was of a stand of deciduous trees, while the other looked out over a blank brick wall. For the purposes of the study, the patient records for both wings were matched in 23 pairs by age, sex, smoking/non-smoking, obesity and so forth. It was found that the tree-view patients spent an average of just under eight days in hospital, whereas the wall-view patients spent almost nine days inside. Additionally, the tree-viewers needed fewer analgesic doses, had fewer negative comments in the nurses' notes and had slightly lower scores for minor post-surgical complications. The author comments wryly that it may not have been that the view of the trees was especially beneficial, but that the blank wall was especially oppressive. Either way, it is clear that a window with a view provided significant therapeutic benefits, and thus should be taken into account at the design stage (Ulrich 1984, 420–421). Building on this work, a team led by Joon-Ho Choi working at the Incheon General Hospital in Korea was able to show that patients recuperating in wards with windows orientated to the sunny south-east recovered faster than those in rooms looking to the shadier north-west. The difference in the average length of stay varied from at least 16% up to as much as 41% in some cases (Choi et al. 2012).

The importance of a room with a view is not just an issue for schools and hospitals: a study published in the *Journal of Environmental Psychology* showed that office workers also need windows for the good of their wellbeing. The work involved three groups of 30 participants who were asked to undertake various tasks in a simulated office setting following on from a low-level stress situation. The three 'offices' were all different: one had a window with a view of greenspace, one had a plasma screen showing a real-time high-definition view of a similar scene, while the third had neither, just a blank wall. Results showed that in terms of heart rate recovery from the low-level stress, the window proved to be more restorative than either of the others, and the more time the participants looked at the window, the more rapidly their heart rate tended to decrease. The plasma worldview therefore had no more benefit than a blank wall in this instance, whereas the window with a real view clearly meant something (Kahn et al. 2008). Similarly, a study conducted in 2011 in a large administrative centre in the University of Oregon suggested that 10% of staff absences could be attributed to those working in offices with no green outlook (Elzeyadi 2011). As for universities, the buildings are often set in spacious grounds, but how often are the students or the academic staff involved in the gardening, planting and maintenance of those landscapes? There are real opportunities here for promoting wellbeing, engaging with nature and developing non-academic but highly educational social interactions.

Greened buildings

But if your office is not located in acres of verdant parkland, there is still a solution: the office itself can be greened by adding indoor plants. After all, as hunter-gatherers we grew up surrounded by plants: a stuffy, sterile indoor environment can certainly be made more visually attractive and more welcoming by their addition. However, they should not be seen as mere ornamentation, since the office greenery will absorb carbon dioxide and emit oxygen while moderating humidity and working to remove volatile organic compounds and other pollutants thrown up by electric equipment, cleaning fluids and synthetic materials. A well-planted office can successfully cure 'sick building syndrome' at the same time as increasing the range of microbiota we all need. It is also suggested that, given the choice, people prefer to work in rooms with plants. They reduce sound and stress levels and improve concentration, plus greened offices have been argued to help reduce absenteeism and aid recovery from mental tiredness.

A study by the University of Exeter conducted during the Chelsea Flower Show in 2013 suggested that staff productivity could be increased by 38%, their creativity by 45% and their wellbeing by 47% with the introduction of suitable plants in appropriate places in and around their workstations. The academics were working with the creative director of Indoor Garden Design, Ian Drummond, who is passionate about "putting living nature into offices", not least because of the health benefits for the workspace. The Chelsea project involved 90 separate experiments and 350 participants working on particular tasks in one of four standard office layouts. Dr Craig Knight, the university psychologist who designed the experiment, observed that the results "indicate that plants, in a well-designed and personalised office environment can boost business effectiveness through improved staff productivity and creativity" (University of Exeter 2013).

These and many other issues are discussed in a major review that is, in part at least, an evolutionary-concordant approach to building design: the World Green Building Council's *Business Case for Green Building* (2013). It argues the case for an environmentally sustainable building industry operating in 98 different countries across the globe, showing how green design and construction methodologies can also save money through reduced energy and maintenance costs and by using less water. It is currently conducting further research into how interior design can improve the workers' wellbeing, an issue with which the studies of the evolutionary determinants of health team can concur (WGBC 2013, 5).

Modern buildings can be designed to be both attractive and effective to work in; older buildings can be reconfigured to keep their character but improve the working environment. The overall message that readers of this book can take home is that, in addition to the issues of social responsibility and duties of care, it simply makes economic sense to design buildings, inside and out, to accommodate the Palaeolithic genome of those who work therein. Unhappy or unhealthy workers are less productive (see www. healthygreenatwork.org, www.greenplantsforgreenbuildings.org).

Home front: designing evolutionary-concordant housing

Greened terraced towns

It is suggested that medium-density, multi-storeyed terraced housing developments of around six storeys will become standard for tomorrow's cities. Families could be housed on the ground and first floors to allow access to a modest urban garden, while balcony flats with one, two or three bedroom multi-occupancy properties could be accessed by stairs if the lift failed, and would not cast too much shadow into the streets below. There is also a case to be made for building on outwards-facing streets (for greater social/tribal interaction), rather than on inward-looking estates (no easy escape route). Other evolutionary determinants would include ready access to outside space as well as the greening of the adjacent streets.

Greened buildings

Since there will not be space for detached villas with gardens front and back for most of the population in the central zones of tomorrow's cities, substantial public parks will be key focal features of the new precincts to increase the biodiversity, microbiota and opportunities for outdoor activities and social interaction. Nevertheless, each flat, maisonette or duplex apartment in the proposed new terraces should be provided with a balcony at least 1.5 m wide or access to a patio or roof terrace, with a minimum of 5 sq. m for each one-bedroom flat, rising by 1–2 sq. m for each extra bedroom. Wherever possible a green roof or green wall should be provided, and ample provision for house plants and window boxes.

Active buildings

Residential blocks should be provided with wide, well-lit staircases to access the upper floors (as well as lifts for those with heavy loads or mobility issues) and secure bicycle storage areas to encourage human locomotion.

Natural light

Glazing for all habitable rooms should be at least 20% of the room area. The living or dining rooms/areas should not be north facing, since they should be able to receive direct sunlight for at least part of each day, and thus should be orientated towards the east, south or west.

Fireplace

Once the open hearth or fireplace was the heart of the home, reflecting the importance of fire to ancient communities. Estate agents will always highlight period features such as open fireplaces when selling older properties; central heating, although more efficient, rarely has the same emotional appeal. Today, the cooker or oven in the open-plan kitchen-diner has become the proxy fire focus for 21st-century city dwellers, subconsciously reflecting its primeval origins.

Domestic buildings

Having briefly commented on offices, schools and hospitals, our attention must turn to domestic buildings, and what form(s) they should take in future urban developments. This discussion starts with the assumption that the cities of the immediate future will be medium to high density, and consequently the notional ideal of a two-storey semi-detached house with front and back gardens is unlikely to be a practical design option for a substantial proportion of urban dwellers. It is clear that tomorrow's new towns will have to incorporate high-density housing, but should that inevitably mean high-rise buildings? Although there are some notable exceptions (such as the Barbican Estate in the City of London, where flats are still eagerly sought after at ever-increasing prices), many of the post-war tower blocks and multi-storeyed estates built in Britain have proved unpopular, impractical and have a layout that often fosters antisocial behaviour. The high costs of construction, maintenance and service charges are rendering them uneconomic, in spite of their engineering innovations and award-winning architecture. Such towers may, nevertheless, have a continuing function as offices, prestigious penthouses, short-term accommodation or pieds-à-terre, but are widely seen as inappropriate for long-term homes.

It must be stressed that there will never be a single building style that suits everyone, since the demands and pockets of young families, extended families, singletons, couples, students, workers on short-term contracts and pensioners will all differ. That said, what are the basic broad principles of residential housing, viewed from a human evolutionary perspective? To open the discussion, it's clear that our Palaeolithic past still impacts on property prices. Any estate agent's valuation will consider the key bread-and-butter elements such as location, access to public transport, size, number of bedrooms and the general condition of the property, plus length of the unexpired lease where appropriate. But man cannot live by bread alone, and for two otherwise identical properties in the same street or same block, there are a number of features which will add (often substantially) to the asking price or the anticipated rental return of one property over another. These unique but evolutionary-determined selling points relate to (a) orientation, windows and view and (b) access to outside space, be it gardens, patios, balconies or terraces. The psychological rationale for this has already been considered in relation to the previous discussion of hospitals, schools and offices (e.g. Ulrich 1984). The economic rationale is simple: a direct view over a river, canal, lake or park can add up to 10% to the price, whereas a beautiful garden in full flower can sell a house on its own. Ideally, the living space should have windows that allow direct sunshine to illuminate the property for at least part of each day. Since such features have been shown to add to our urban wellbeing, we are consequently prepared to pay a premium for them. But should not one of the objectives for the next generation of cities be how to incorporate such welcome features into new residential developments as standard?

As to the question of human scale in large housing developments, it was once suggested that an intuitive mathematics test might resolve the problem of when a building is too tall: most humans can tell at a glance whether a building is one to four storeys high – they don't have to count the windows. However, with tower blocks you can't differentiate between a 14- or a 18-storey tower unless you actually count the windows. While accepting that the view from a penthouse on the 25th floor might be stunning, as a general guideline, a maximum six-storey building could be a more human model to work with for relatively high-density residential occupation.

Polytribal architecture

The author once lived in a ground-floor flat with a tiny inner-city patio some 4 m x 5 m backing on to communal urban greenspace. It was visited at various times of the day and night by creatures from many different tribes. Not all got on with each other (indeed, death threats were commonplace), but every day saw the same procession. Squirrels arrived early to see if any nuts had been left out; birds came and went throughout the day, seeking seeds or insects; cats patrolled and sunned themselves in the afternoon when the weather was beneficent; foxes passed through at night, scouring the area for whatever such scavengers could find. In other words, all made use of the same small urban space, sometimes tolerating each other, sometimes avoiding each other. All saw it as part of 'their' territory even if, according to the land registry, it legally belonged to me (although was financially still owned by a mortgage company). This seems an interesting analogy for the development of 'shared space initiatives', where sections of road are no longer so clearly segregated for pedestrians, cyclists and cars: all the groups have to negotiate their way along/across the route with as few incidents as possible. Rather than being directed by traffic lights and road signs, all the travellers have to use their eyes, ears and common sense to complete their journey on a shared surface.

In a similar way, a town has many stakeholders with different perspectives and thus incorporates many tribes (as described in Chapter 8). Diversity will certainly be the norm in tomorrow's largest cities; while it might be hard for everybody to embrace all of it – given various inevitable conflicts of interest – at least, like the patio in Hackney or on the shared space projects in Poynton town, Cheshire, the various tribes passing through it can be aware of each other's space and be tolerant of their differing needs.

The larger the conurbation, the more tribes there will be – culturally, geographically, professionally, socially. As we saw in Chapter 9, Professor Dunbar has suggested that most of us can only cope psychologically with some 150 friends and relations, a figure which can be associated with the size of our earliest hunter-gatherer societies. Culturally, most city dwellers will be polytribal – that is, they will belong to several different tribes simultaneously. We can identify with a particular social class, our immediate neighbours, our work colleagues or wider professional affiliations, we can be supporters of a football team (usually just one) and have a shared national identity, faith or political creed; all these groupings serve as 'tribes', and our behaviour and persona may actually differ, depending on which of these tribes we are with at any one time. And it is this polytribal phenomenon, a relatively modern cultural adaption, that lies at the heart of successful (or unsuccessful) urban living with its necessarily complex social interactions.

Based on the most simplistic interpretation of our hunter-gatherer past, we could suggest that modern towns should be designed as a series of modular, self-contained communities (i.e. tribes), laid out around the urban civic centre like planets around the sun, a system that is not dissimilar to the network of connected settlements suggested by Sir Ebenezer Howard. Such an approach also resonates with the New Urbanists' approach to the building and connecting of 'traditional neighbourhoods'. Such units certainly meet the requirements of families and local school catchment areas, and the needs of those particular tribal groups can be (and often are) addressed architecturally through considered town planning.

But the often conflicting and changing needs of the many other urban tribes (e.g. the shifting populations of itinerant workers, students or singletons who don't require ready access to primary schools) are often less easy to embed in the town plan. They require a rather more fluid and flexible approach to building size and type. Our polytribal cities need to be architecturally multi-layered and multi-used, and that is a challenge in itself. However, if lorries, car drivers and pedestrians can share sections of the road, as some notable examples have shown, then there is hope for a polytribal urban fabric.

Remaking the city: evolutionary-concordant retrofits

We have discussed a set of features for any city which genuinely wishes to accommodate our Palaeolithic genome. The catalogue includes fresh air and fresh water, medium-rise housing with large windows and outside space, active office buildings, traffic-calmed greened streets, a network of designated cycle routes and walkways integrated with an effective public transport system, parks, sporting facilities, city farms, allotments and community gardens. That long list could be set alongside the "characteristics of Paleo places" suggested by Elizabeth Rodriguez in her 2015 study of town planning from a human evolutionary perspective, *Paleo Places* (pers. com.). These include the basic need for grasslands, open water, clear vistas and the evidence of food. All these elements could work together to provide a cohesive structural and social semi-lattice, to adopt the terminology used by the architect Christopher Alexander (1965). To mount such an evolutionary-concordant retrofit of a city would provide it with a system that both underpins and promotes positive urban wellbeing. And many cities already promote some or most of these features, but often as separate initiatives emanating from different offices within the same local planning authority, borough or council, perhaps responding to demands from a higher transport, health or regional planning body. A better understanding of the biology behind clever urban design should lead to a more coordinated programme that recognises the significance and major benefits of an evolutionary-concordant approach: cities fit for humans. The town may not be our natural habitat, but we can make it our optimal one.

Chapter 15

REVELATIONS

Savage renaissance

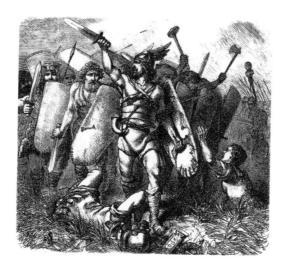

Figure 15.1. Noble savages: this tribe defeated the civilised Roman army.

In 1877, Lewis Morgan published a seven-stage progress model for mankind, beginning with Lower Savagery (a culture of gathering), moving through Middle and Upper Savagery (with fishing, fire and bows and arrows), progressing to Lower and Middle Barbarism (pottery, plant and animal husbandry) and Upper Barbarism (metalworking), until Civilisation is finally reached with the invention of writing (Morgan 1877, 9–19). His endearingly politically incorrect terminology sharply focuses on the underlying concepts and value judgements which tacitly persist in much of our modern thinking: mankind was moving along a predestined path to become more and more civilised, so prehistory was merely the prelude, our infancy, before we finally grew up (e.g. Pluciennik 2005). It is undeniable that there has been an astonishing transformation in society over the last few millennia, but was it inevitable? Is that what the gods dictated our fate should be? Is 'progress' just an optimistic word for 'change', or is all change progress?

But will we ever be able to uncivilise the detrimental effects of urbanisation on our wellbeing? Some have argued that modernity was prefaced by the Renaissance, which saw a rebirth of learning and art based on the rediscovery of the wisdom of the ancients from the Mediterranean classical world. Is it too fanciful to suggest that the regeneration of urbanism in the 21st century could be based upon a new Renaissance, the rediscovery of our uncivilised Palaeolithic genome, a robust legacy more ancient than Aristotle? Certainly, the awful rise in lifestyle diseases that has accompanied recent urbanisation must be addressed, since cities are forever expanding, and by far the largest proportion of the global population will be living in towns for the foreseeable future. If we are to live healthy (i.e. normal) lives in the artificial environment we have created for ourselves, then something has to change. Real progress in 21st-century social evolution seems to demand a return to simulated versions of Morgan's Lower, Middle and Upper Savagery.

If the adoption of the protocols described below could be shown to eradicate, or at least contain, the unwelcome physiological, psychological and societal aspects of current urbanisation, then surely that would be seen as a positive adaption: it would create an urban gene pool that could better cope with modernity, and was thus finally fit for purpose.

Build a better zoo

We have seen that the town is not our natural habitat: in human evolutionary terms, it's a recent settlement type that has only been developing over the last 5,000 to 10,000 years, and it's still changing. Indeed, modern cities are highly complex entities, responsive to powerful economic forces and political factors which operate and interact on local, regional and global scales: change is therefore inevitable. By contrast, although *Homo sapiens* has seen major cultural developments since the Stone Age, our physiology and psychology have remained much as they were for a million years or more when life was lived in the wild. In a true evolutionary sense, the urbanised human race seems like a fish out of water. We weren't designed to live in towns, but that's where we will all end up. In 2012, the United Nations Department of Economic and Social Affairs predicted a major phase of urban expansion in which the global population living in cities will double in just 40 years to a staggering 6.3 billion people (UN-DESA 2012, 1). Architecture group Terreform One's Mitchell Joachim has commented that, rather than describing the current era as the Anthropocene, it could be more correctly termed the 'Capitalocene', since our economies, culture and society are now all urban based (see Anderson 2016).

Building towns and expanding cities for an extra three billion people will happen; indeed, is already happening. But beneath the architecture of the new towns, beneath the plans, the challenges and the suggested solutions lie the humans who have to live there, work there and move around there. Unless the next generations of urban settlements are designed, first and foremost, as healthy cities and are built for humans (that is to say, on evolutionary-concordant lines), we will have constructed our very own urban wellbeing crisis on a truly global scale, and one that may spiral beyond the control of public health authorities. Western lifestyle diseases can be designed out of the plans for tomorrow's world, if we so choose.

The zoologist and sociobiologist Desmond Morris likened human urban life to that of animals caged in a zoo: certainly there are benefits to modern civilisation, but there are also costs, as *The Human Zoo* describes (Morris 1969). For some the solution has been to reject modern society, technology and towns altogether and return to a rural regime of subsistence living. Alas, with a world population approaching eight billion, there is not enough room for everybody to take that option. The approach proposed in this study is a more practical compromise: urban life can be significantly improved if society re-embraces at least some of the cardinal concepts of its half-forgotten former life. If we could reconfigure personal lives, townscapes and urban society by progressing, rather than suppressing, a raft of innate evolutionary attributes, then town life and town lives will be materially improved.

To counter the reinvention of the slums of tomorrow, we should focus on the naked apes that will live in tomorrow's cities, and reconfigure townscapes that offer them at least a flavour of their natural habitat. An evolutionary-concordant town can integrate the real advantages of modernity with the unbending demands of our evolutionary legacy. After all, since a town is a human creation, it can be changed, modified or reconfigured: the form(s) it takes on in the future – short or long term – lies in our hands. We can therefore choose *not* to construct towns more suited to our biology, our inherited Palaeolithic genome, towns that do not accommodate the human evolutionary determinants of health, social behaviour and our necessary 'genetic responses' to nature. Or we can take the conscious decision to build a better zoo.

Eden Protocol

Lifestyle choices are moulded by a complex of cultural, economic and societal influences. The research summarised in this book has incorporated studies concerning physiological, metabolic and psychological factors relating to nutrition, activity regimes and social interactions. But by no means do all such choices lead to personal or social wellbeing in the longer term. The Alameda County Study was undertaken by the epidemiologist Sir Richard Doll, in which a cluster of lifestyle factors were related over time to a higher or lower risk of death: these were termed 'positive' and 'negative' health behaviours. In a similar vein, the evolutionary determinants of health programme has identified 'normal' evolutionary-concordant behaviours as well as 'abnormal' non-evolutionary-concordant behaviours. Despite significant achievements over the previous century, it is now evident that modern medicine on its own cannot solve all health problems: its resources are over-stretched and its limitations increasingly recognised. Significant progress is no longer solely a matter of eradicating particular diseases, but requires an improved understanding of the political, economic, cultural, social and genetic determinants of health. To improve a nation's wellbeing must now rely not just on medical advances but also on positive cultural and behavioural change. The interdisciplinary programme described in this book aims to make a contribution to that debate not just through the identification and consideration of key physiological, psychological and societal determinants, but also to suggest directions for the formulation of policies and practices that could translate directly into improved urban wellbeing.

In the past, public health officials and town planners worked together in the drive to eradicate such urban evils as cholera and typhoid. One of the prime goals for the new generation of cities must be an equally concerted drive to improve urban wellbeing, as the expanding Healthy Cities movement shows. The concepts underlying the evolutionary determinants of health programme could have a major role in that work, realigning policy and practice to better fit our biology. It would be far more cost effective to work with our Palaeolithic genome rather than continuing the losing battle to maintain a lifestyle that is fundamentally bad for us.

Although town life is, superficially, the very antithesis of the hunter-gatherers' world, this urban paradox can be at least partially resolved. A solution lies in the adoption of proxy behaviours, environments and townscapes that mimic key elements of the nutrition, daily activity, social interaction and engagement with the natural world that our minds and bodies demand consciously, unconsciously or subconsciously. Positive attributes of this shared evolutionary past need to be developed, while negative elements must be constrained. The practices that such applications suggest have been brought together to form a coherent protocol applied to

21st-century townscapes and urban lifestyles. We call this approach the Eden Protocol, a short-hand term for the evolutionary determinants of health, social behaviour and urban wellbeing.

We have discussed in detail how our Palaeolithic genome still has influence on our everyday urban lives. The impact on our wellbeing can be positive if we build on that biology, or negative if we decide to override it. Under the banner of the Eden Protocol, a series of guidelines have been drawn up to progress this concept (summarised in the box 'Evolutionary concordance'). Unsurprisingly, many of the elements in the Personal Protocol appear in healthy living guidance issued by public health authorities across the globe, but usually without the Palaeolithic perspective. A more overt evolutionary focus on such advice appears increasingly in lifestyle literature from the Primal movement in California (e.g. Sissons 2009) to academics in Europe (e.g. Heylighen 2010). In this book, however, the scope is considerably widened, presenting evidence-based research to support the case not just for reconfiguring our lifestyles (a very good place to start) but also our buildings and even our town plans.

Evolutionary concordance

The Eden Protocol incorporates suggestions (not statutory impositions) on how modern-day urban living can better fit our biology – our uncivilised genes – and thus significantly improve our wellbeing. There is clearly some overlap between these lists: some individuals might be tempted to go it alone, perhaps to take up cycling as their daily commute (Personal Protocol), but encouragement and support in the workplace would obviously be beneficial: a covered cycle rack, for example (Employer Protocol). Then again, the more your city had designated cycle tracks stripped of heavy lorries turning left, the more likely you would be to cycle (Urban Design Protocol). But what comes first: the chicken or the egg, the bike or the designated cycle track?

Personal Protocol

This is a summary of the key themes in a health behaviour package that most individuals can have, or can develop, control over. Most are based on aspects of a hunter-gatherer lifestyle reworked for a 21st-century context. It is not seen as an evolutionary regression but as a return to a normality in keeping with our biology. The first half of the protocol looks at 'good health', which equates with a lifestyle in which our physiology functions normally in an evolutionary-concordant fashion. Should we repeatedly or continuously indulge in abnormal (i.e.

non-evolutionary-concordant) behaviours, then 'poor health' will ultimately ensue. The second half of the list looks at features that relate to 'happiness', a 21st-century concept that is evolutionary concordant on a psychological level, but refined and balanced by legality and modern cultural mores. It includes the need to be challenged, take risks and be prepared to push yourself – essential attributes in the uncertain world of the hunter-gatherer.

- Eat healthily.

- Walk or cycle all or part of the way to school/work/college whenever possible.

- Use stairs, rather than lifts, whenever possible.

- Limit smoking and alcohol consumption.

- Take an active part in the life of your family or household.

- Take an active part in the convivial social life of your community through, for example, sport, music, engagement with nature or a range of other social activities.

- Spend as much time out of doors as the weather permits, preferably in greenspace or at least greened streets.

- Challenge yourself physically and mentally.

- Take an active interest in your town, its past, its present and its future.

It should not need stressing that enjoying normal health is an important factor in promoting wellbeing, and thus many of the items listed here can be profitably integrated. You could, for example, eat a healthy outdoor picnic with friends and family in a place you had not previously visited. That would represent an excellent evolutionary-concordant day out, especially if it involved a walk up the hill to get there (and the English weather might also add a further character-building challenge).

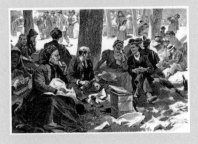

Quality of life: eating al fresco with family and friends.

Working from the themes described in the Personal Protocol above, the next three sections look at the responsibilities of our employers, our schools and our universities, and suggest how these bodies might encourage and facilitate positive health behaviours for their staff and students. The lists are not exhaustive: they can be added to by more creative employers.

University Protocol

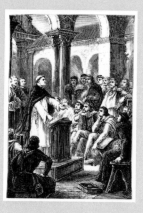

Learning by degrees: a medieval education.

- Ensure healthy, nutritious food and drink is provided in the refectory.

- Discourage the sale of unhealthy foods/drinks (e.g. those with added sugars).

- Encourage active commuting to/from university for staff and students.

- Provide sufficient cycle racks, lockers and showers.

- Encourage the use of stairs rather than lifts for all those able to do so.

- Discourage over-sedentary work patterns.

- Ensure as many courses as possible have field-trip/external element(s).

- Ensure lectures where students are seated do not last beyond one hour without a break.

- Provide sports facilities.

- Promote and facilitate music, dancing and sport for all, regardless of degree subject.

- Provide attractive public open spaces, suitably planted and maintained.

- Encourage student participation in campus gardening.

- Provide and maintain plants within the buildings, wherever appropriate.

- Encourage student participation in their tending (at least in term time).

School Protocol

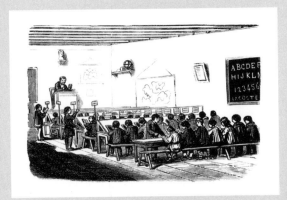

Class act.

- Ensure healthy, nutritious food and drink is provided on the premises.

- Discourage the sale of unhealthy foods/drinks (e.g. those with added sugars) in or near the school.

- Encourage walking/cycling to/from school for pupils and teachers.

- Provide sufficient cycle racks and lockers.

- Encourage use of stairs rather than lifts for all those able to do so.

- Discourage over-sedentary work patterns.

- Ensure that all classes spend at least 25% of each day outside the classroom.

- Provide facilities that actively promote team sports, individual sports and general exercise.

- Promote and facilitate music and dancing within the weekly curriculum for all.

- Provide and maintain plants within the buildings, wherever appropriate.

- Encourage pupil participation in gardening/looking after plants and animals.

- Ensure all pupils are challenged academically and physically.

Employer Protocol

- Ensure healthy, nutritious food and drink is provided in the canteen.

- Discourage the sale of unhealthy foods/drinks (e.g. those with added sugars).

- Encourage active commuting.

- Provide sufficient cycle racks, lockers and showers.

- Encourage use of stairs rather than lifts for all those able to do so.

- Develop new work patterns and office layouts for staff in the most sedentary roles.

- Provide and maintain plants within the buildings, wherever appropriate.

- Encourage staff participation in their tending.

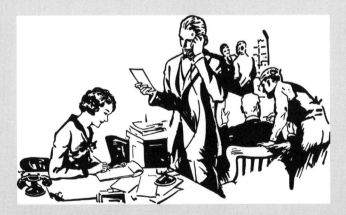

Working lives.

The final section suggests approaches open to local authorities and planning agencies that can facilitate urban wellbeing, providing a safe, healthy, greened infrastructure and a good standard of building and public realm provision. It is a hybrid of similar thinking developed quite independently by, for example, the Healthy Cities movement and New Urbanists, with a 21st-century revision of some of Sir Ebenezer Howard's thinking on garden cities. Consideration of the evolutionary determinants of health provides an integrated rationale underpinning those initiatives.

Urban Design Protocol

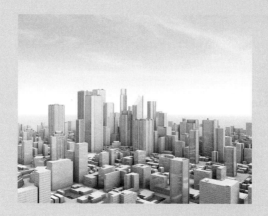

The way forward or urban nightmare?

- Provide fresh water and sound sanitation systems.

- Ensure good air quality (e.g. limit or ban vehicles that emit diesel particulates).

- Put human locomotion at the heart of transport policy and street design (e.g. traffic-calming measures, designated cycle tracks, pedestrianisation).

- Develop an integrated public transport system that helps to limit car use.

- Develop designated cycle and pedestrian route-ways.

- Maintain or extend urban greenspace.

- Promote and develop participatory urban greenspace (e.g. allotments, community gardens, city farms).

- Promote sport through the development of pitches, sports facilities, etc.

- Develop programmes of street greening.

- Promote the development of roof gardens etc.

- Limit development of high-rise buildings for residential use (maximum six storeys preferable).

- Encourage street-based neighbourhoods rather than enclosed estates.

- Ensure residential buildings have adequate natural light.

- Ensure all residential units have access to some outside space (garden, patio, terrace or balcony).

Adopting deep behavioural change (AD/BC)

So how might these protocols become more widely adopted? First, there is spreading the word, hoping that by reading or hearing about our Palaeolithic genome's relevance to the 21st century, the protocols discussed in this book will be put into active service. Publication is but an essential first step: a back-up plan will also be required. This is a whole new programme still being developed that goes under the umbrella term AD/BC, an acronym for adopting deep behavioural change. Our hunter-gatherer psyche is not based solely on reason and logic, but is just as open to intuition and emotion when it comes to decision-making. Ask any politician seeking election how many votes are won by those who write the manifesto, and how many by the spin doctors and image consultants? It's difficult to persuade people to alter their behaviour just by being reasonable; if it were that simple, there would be no smoking, obesity-related illness or religious bigotry. There has to be a raft of approaches including celebrity endorsement, new legislation, cost benefits, media campaigns and town planning initiatives.

The alchemy of behavioural change (NICE 2007) concerns just such a complex lattice of social and urban planning, fiscal measures, education and incentivisation, coercion and legislation (Michie et al. 2014). The first stage would be to identify the scope and scale of each particular challenge to be addressed, and then the target group that would most benefit from a change, before the means to effect the desired modifications can be designed. Take an example from Denmark, where a study examined the relationship between dietary patterns, demography and health-related lifestyle factors

(Knudsen et al. 2014). The team worked from data collected for a national survey of adults over the period 2003–2008. The study identified three clear demographic dietary patterns:

1. The 'fast-food group' consuming pizza, hamburgers, crisps, rice and pasta, sugar-sweetened soft drinks and sweets tended to be younger and were more likely to be smokers.

2. The 'traditional group' consuming rye bread, white bread, cheese, jam, cold meat, minced meat, potatoes and gravy, cake and biscuits were usually male and usually older.

3. The 'health-conscious group' consuming coarse bread, fruit, vegetables, low-fat dairy, nuts, water and tea were mainly female and had a better educational level.

Such basic research is essential for targeting future nutritional education at those considered most at risk. It could be argued that in Denmark, that would be Group 1, and thus advertising strategies could be focused on them in a cost-effective and health-effective manner.

Similar studies in the UK have highlighted an alarming rise in obesity in schoolchildren, where in 2015, nearly 30% of those aged 2 to 15 were classed as obese or overweight, according to Public Health England (see http://www.noo.org.uk/NOO_about_obesity/child_obesity). As a consequence, the National Institute for Health and Care Excellence have recommended that local planning authorities should consider restricting planning permission for takeaway and fast-food outlets within walking distance of schools. A report by Dr Nick Cavill and Professor Harry Rutter was then published by Public Health England in 2013. This provided the background to the problem and set out the ways in which local authorities could take appropriate action to effect behaviour change both through improved education and within the townscape itself.

Evolutionary-concordant urbanisation

So what might be the impact on a new urban population if there was widespread adoption of these personal and institutional protocols, encouraged by living in a city with active buildings set in an evolutionary-concordant town plan? Possible answers might be suggested by consideration of Table 15.1 below, a revised version of Table 1.1. The first column presents the most common causes of death in the un-urbanised community of Kitava, with the ten most common causes of death in urbanising and highly urbanised population in columns 2 and 3 respectively. Note how, as one set of diseases or conditions is contained during the process of urbanisation (columns 2–3), their place in the world rankings is taken by another. It's clear that lessons learned by modern medical research and robust public health programmes have proved their worth, removing, for example, causes of infant mortality from column 3. This proves that significant progress in improving urban wellbeing is demonstrably possible, given sufficient political will.

It is often argued that populations live progressively longer lives on average as they become increasingly urbanised, and thus the top ten killers in an urbanised society could be seen as a catalogue of the inevitable diseases and conditions of old age: the older we live, the more likely it is that we will suffer and die from one of them. But there is an alternative view. Supposing that the evolutionary-concordant lessons to be learned from the positive health behaviours embedded in the daily lives of hunter-gatherers (or modern proxy-hunter-gatherers) were adopted more widely, that situation could significantly impact on mortality rates and health profiles by removing the urbanised column's leading causes from the equation, or at least containing them. Perhaps simple 'old age' could become the most common cause of death in our 21st-century urban future?

Might tomorrow's evolutionary-concordant cities combine the health benefits of evolutionary-concordant non-urbanised communities (by keeping these rare causes of death rare) with those of our contemporary urbanised communities?

Table 15.1. New world order

	Evolutionary-concordant non-urbanised	Urbanising	Non-evolutionary-concordant urbanised	Evolutionary-concordant urbanised
Old age	Y	Y	Y	Y
Accidents/homicide	Y			?
Neonatal infections	Y	8th		?
Malarial infections etc.	Y	9th		?
Prematurity/low birth weight	Y	10th		?
Diarrhoeal disease	N	3rd		?
HIV	N	4th		?

	Evolutionary-concordant non-urbanised	Urbanising	Non-evolutionary-concordant urbanised	Evolutionary-concordant urbanised
Tuberculosis	N	7th		?
Coronary heart disease	N	2nd	1st	?
Stroke/cerebrovascular disease	N	5th	2nd	?
Trachea/bronchus/lung cancer	N		3rd	?
Lower respiratory infections	N	1st	4th	?
Chronic obstructive pulmonary disease	N	6th	5th	?
Alzheimer's/dementia	N		6th	?
Colon/rectum cancers	N		7th	?
Diabetes	N		8th	?
Breast cancer	N		9th	?
Stomach cancer	N		10th	?

Sources: Lindeberg 2010, 58–63, 102–103, 116–119, 134, 157–160; Ridsdale and Gallop 2010, table 4.1.

Aligning our personal health behaviours more closely with our biology is simply playing to our strengths, allowing our physiology, metabolism and immune systems to operate at maximum efficiency. But modern conurbations and cultures also need to be realigned to support such endeavours, and this concerns not just individuals but civic authorities, governments, commerce, industry and agriculture. The following examples show how a raft of personal and institutional lifestyle changes, together with evolutionary-concordant urban design (i.e. integrating all our Eden Protocols), could help to ensure that our current major causes of mortality would not feature in the list for tomorrow's world (column 4).

To begin with, while not decrying or downplaying the successes achieved by pharmaceutical treatments or medical interventions in the fight against cancers, consider the significant role that our robust but uncivilised genes can also play in this battle. A major study in the United States consulted the health records of approximately 136,000 adults, divided into two cohorts. One cohort, the low-risk group of 16,531 women and 11,731 men, enjoyed a broadly evolutionary-concordant lifestyle: this was defined as maintaining a BMI of 18.5–25 (a reflection of 'normal' nutritional and activity regimes), doing at least two and a half hours of moderate exercise regularly each week, not smoking and consuming no more than two alcoholic drinks a day (male) or one a day (female). As for the remaining 73,040 women and 34,608 men, their profiles did not match all four of those criteria, and they were thus considered the high-risk group. When the incidence and mortality of total and major individual carcinomas in the two groups was compared, dramatic differences were recorded. From this it was argued that a substantial cancer burden would be prevented simply through lifestyle modification. Precisely how dramatic that difference would be was shown when these figures were extrapolated to the entire US population. If there was a widespread adoption of broadly evolutionary-concordant lifestyles, deaths from lung cancer could be slashed by 80%, bowel cancer up to 30%, prostate cancer by 21% and breast cancer by 12% (Song and Giovannucci 2016).

As yet more countries urbanise ever more intensively, a positive pandemic of obesity is developing (Popkin et al. 2012). Modern urban living has witnessed a massive increase in a range of lifestyle diseases such as type 2 diabetes. It has been suggested that our bodies and metabolism once responded to periods of scarcity with an insulin response that enabled fat deposits to be stored. Today, even though our food supplies are far less erratic, our uncivilised genes are still thriftily conserving those fats, unaware of the damage they are inflicting on us (Neel 1962). David Napier, UCL professor of medical anthropology, is studying the global incidence of diabetes, set to rise from 415 million to 642 million cases by 2040. His conclusion is that it is not just unhealthy diets and sedentary behaviour driving the rise, but the very process of urbanisation itself. Two-thirds of diabetics live in towns, and that figure is anticipated to increase dramatically as countries such as China and India accelerate their industrialisation programmes. His research with diabetics in Copenhagen, Houston, Mexico City, Shanghai and Tianjin is developing policies to break the link between diabetes and such unnatural urbanisation (see UCL 2015). There is, of course, a societal dimension that also needs to be addressed. Jonathan Wells is the professor of anthropology and paediatric nutrition at the UCL Institute of Child Health. In his study, *The Metabolic Ghetto*, he discusses why particular social groups are more impacted by obesity, diabetes, hypertension and cardiovascular disease than others. His ground-breaking work integrates physiological, evolutionary, nutritional, economic and societal perspectives, demonstrating both the complexity of the challenge and the possible solutions (Wells 2016).

To this must be added the continuing debate on the relative merits of differ-ing treatments for obesity and type 2 diabetes. These range from metabolic surgery (e.g. the fitting of gastric bands: see Rubino et al. 2016), pharmaceu-tical products and behavioural interventions, such as adopting evolutionary-concordant nutritional and activity regimes. As for the latter, a report published by the American Diabetes Association in January 2016 showed strong and consistent evidence that progression from pre-diabetes to type 2 diabetes can be delayed by supervised lifestyle interventions. In addi-tion, these approaches (e.g. diet, physical activity and behavioural therapy) can also prove beneficial in the actual treatment of type 2 diabetes for over-weight and obese patients. This can be achieved through weight-loss programmes offering a 500–750 kcal/day energy deficit or providing 1,250–1,500 kcal/day for women and 1,750–2,000 kcal/day for men, adjusted for the individual's baseline body weight (American Diabetes Association 2016). For some patients, depending on the severity of their condition, surgical or pharmaceutical treatments may still be the preferred treatment, but for many, there is now clear evidence that lifestyle interven-tions – that is, a return to more 'normal' dietary and activity regimes – also offer the possibility of containment or cure.

As for our urban design protocols, it is argued here that town plans should encourage human locomotion. If our streets, parks and buildings genuinely facilitate active lives, then it has been estimated that, just in London, more than 4,000 premature deaths, nearly 800 more cases of breast cancer, up to 500 more cases of colorectal cancer, 1,500 extra cases of coronary heart disease and nearly 45,000 more cases of type 2 diabetes could be avoided (TfL 2014, 75).

A long drawn-out battle for our health that requires regulation, legislation and changes to production processes is, of course, the addition of sugars to industrially prepared foods and drinks. Admittedly, the responsibility for what we eat is primarily personal. Nevertheless, the continued production and marketing of foodstuffs that destroy teeth and contribute directly to obesity when consumed in quantity arguably incorporates a measure of corporate irresponsibility. We can try sugar taxes and dramatic labelling highlighting ingredients and consequences, but changing the recipe and the culture would have greater impact in the long return journey back to nor-mality for our un-urbanised digestive systems.

We also now know that smoking is a killer, but it has taken a long and hard-fought struggle against vested interests to persuade people to give it up or not to start that non-evolutionary-concordant addiction. We have, in theory at least, some personal responsibility regarding whether or not we smoke, but it is not just tobacco that poses such a fatal risk to our respiratory system: the very urban air we breathe can kill us, and that is something we as indi-viduals have far less control over. In June 2016, the Mayors of London and

Paris, Sadiq Khan and Anne Hidalgo, wrote to the European Union's Environment Council demanding tough and legally binding targets to address the continent's low air quality. The dreadful statistics spoke for themselves, but only for those who were prepared to listen. Every year, some 400,000 people across Europe die as a consequence of their long-term exposure to air pollution. Current testing proposals for pollutants emitted from vehicles are often not rigorous enough to successfully meet this challenge, while the infamous Volkswagen emissions scandal demonstrates how far car manufacturers will go to deliberately falsify test results. The use of chemical weapons on civilian populations is now classified as a war crime, but many of the most polluting vehicles are still not banned on our city streets; indeed, it may take until 2030 to agree and implement rigorous and effective emission limits for key air pollutants. Alas, our lungs have still not evolved sufficiently to adapt to poor urban air quality. If we, or our children, are ever to enjoy fresh air in our towns, it will take time, new legislation and dramatic changes in vehicle design, use and numbers. For several thousand people, that change will come too late.

Bringing together all these studies, a case can therefore be made for the suggestion that most of the top ten causes of death in modern highly urbanised societies (see Table 15.1, column 3) are not an inevitable consequence of old age, but are largely premature deaths – an inevitable consequence of non-evolutionary-concordant urbanisation and non-evolutionary-concordant lifestyles.

Urban adaptions

To sum up, it has been shown that we have evolved culturally far, far faster than we have evolved genetically: our Palaeolithic genome remains largely unchanged, un-urbanised and uncivilised. We can't change it, but we can change our culture and our townscapes to better accommodate the immutable evolutionary determinants of health and social behaviour. Reconfiguring our lives, our buildings, our streets and our urban societies is a big ask, but it also brings a big result: significantly improved urban wellbeing. By adopting the suggested protocols, this book has suggested what might be done through individual endeavour, by supportive employers and forward-thinking urban designers, all with the support of local and national governments and their agencies. It also demonstrates why it should be done: it's not that adopting the Eden Protocol is good for us, it's just that *not* adopting the Eden Protocol is bad for us, since it leads to an unstoppable rise in obesity, diabetes, cardiovascular disease, allergenic disorders, antisocial behaviours, costs to the National Health Service – the litany goes on. The choice is ours, and various ways that we can begin to adapt our culture and our behaviour for the better have been proposed.

Towns are not our natural habitat. That said, *Homo sapiens* has demonstrated that it is nothing if not adaptable: it has colonised virtually every corner of the terrestrial planet and subsequently gone on to domesticate plants, animals and half its own species in its unprecedented population explosion. Its next global challenge, the next battleground, is the housing and support of an extra two billion souls in the next 30 years. This will take urbanisation to an undreamt-of level. If we are to survive and prosper in such an extended artificial environment, then we will need all the help and direction we can get. We must pay heed to our robust and ancient genes. They may be uncivilised, but they have already proved their worth by underpinning the survival of mankind for millennia.

Tomorrow's cities and tomorrow's urban societies would be much healthier if configured or reconfigured on evolutionary-concordant principles. Life in such a city would, by definition, be so much easier, working with our Palaeolithic genome rather than against it. The human race has adapted to living in the forest, the valleys, the desert, the jungle, the mountains and the open plains. But can it take the next step in its evolutionary progress, and adapt rather more successfully to an extensive urban environment of its own making? Towns may not be our natural habitat, but we can make them our optimal one.

EPILOGUE

Uncivilised enlightenment

While writing this book I noticed how often many unrelated bodies following different lines of enquiry had reached similar conclusions as to the potency of the evolutionary determinants of health, social behaviour and urban design. Although most had little concept of the underpinning deep genetic imperatives, all could see positive results. These included the caring professions studying the therapeutic impact that gardening, keeping pets or music can have; organic farmers and nutritionists calculating the recommended daily allowance of fruit and vegetables; health professionals constructing beneficial activity regimes as well as the walkers and cyclists who had long practised them; social workers looking at the positive benefits of sport in urban areas; poets pondering the deeper meaning of love, life and hosts of golden daffodils; politicians debating their constituents' happiness and wellbeing; the National Health Service contemplating the ever-rising costs of the obesity epidemic; architects designing homes and buildings for humans; community groups pressing for better streetscapes; town planners working with public health officials; urban designers who value greenspace; and preservationists and activists fighting to save cherished environments. For all those, and for many more who are trying to make urbanisation work, perhaps a better understanding of our shared deep past will materially assist the construction of a more normal, healthier future. Indeed, it is suggested here that the unifying paradigm underpinning all these varied initiatives is the wider and deeper concept of evolutionary concordance.

Remaking modernity

Towns are an artificial creation, and thus they are an environment over which we can have some control. Many more are being built to accommodate an expanding global urban population that will reach six billion by 2050. We can remake modernity in such a way that it better reflects our biology, or we can consciously choose not to. The lessons of human evolutionary archaeology should be central to the reconfiguration of urban lifestyles and for planning the next generation of cities: if we are ever to adapt more successfully to them, then tomorrow's mega-urban landscapes should be based on evolutionary-concordant designs.

This book has evaluated not only relevant nutritional and activity regimes, but it has also considered changes in town plans, building design, urban greenspace, the school and university curriculum, food production and processing and, following the Volkswagen emissions scandal, car manufacture and use. Such an agenda on its own will not, of course, replace such established initiatives as the social determinants of health programme or that of the Healthy Cities movement, but it could underpin, facilitate and actively complement them. All in all, a modest cultural revolution has been suggested in which evolutionary-concordant behaviours become the new norm for urban wellbeing. But this is just a book. It is pointedly not a political manifesto, or a philosophical tract or a religious mantra. It is an expression of a point of view, for which supporting evidence-based research has been presented. Some would argue that it's just common sense. Alas, it's not always common practice (yet).

APPENDIX 1: HUNTER-GATHERERS WITH LATITUDE

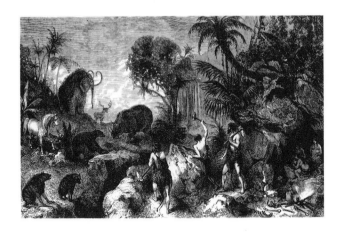

Living with nature: an idealised image of a hunter-gatherer community.

What does the term 'hunter-gatherer' actually mean? In *The Lifeways of Hunter-Gatherers*, Professor Robert Kelly tabulates the dietary range of 126 hunter-gatherer communities that survived into the modern era, shown with an approximate percentage of the food they derived from hunting, gathering and/or fishing (Kelly 2013, 40, table 3). Those data are reworked in the new summary table below, showing just a selection of the very different regimes presented, subdivided and ranked according to the principal food groups consumed.

The geographical zones occupied by these tribes range from the Arctic to the tropics, and these widely differing environments are denoted by the figure representing the effective temperature (ET) of the region (i.e. the mean of the coldest and hottest months). The range runs from 8 at the poles to 26 at the equator; low ET values represent cold environments with short growing seasons, while the higher ET values include tropical habitats with long growing seasons. Note how the dietary regimes change with latitude (i.e. as ET values increase) reflecting the changing environments occupied.

Hunter-gatherers, fisher-hunters or gatherer-hunters?

FISHER-HUNTER (ET 8.7–10.5)	*Hunt*	*Gather*	*Fish*
Tagiugmiut (Tareumiut) ET 8.7	30%	0	**70%**
Angmagsalik ET 9.0	20%	0	**80%**
Copper Inuit ET 9.1	40%	0	**60%**
Baffinland Inuit ET 9.3	5%	0	**95%**
Chugach Inuit ET 10.5	20%	0	**80%**
FISHER-HUNTER-GATHERER (ET 8.5–12.7)	*Hunt*	*Gather*	*Fish*
Polar Inuit ET 8.5	40%	10%	**50%**
Sivokakhmeit ET 9.0	15%	5%	**80%**
Nunivak ET 10.9	30%	10%	**60%**
Saulteaux ET 11.7	35%	20%	**45%**
Alsea ET 12.7	20%	10%	**70%**
FISHER-GATHERER-HUNTER (ET 12.4–18.3)	*Hunt*	*Gather*	*Fish*
Shuswap ET 12.4	30%	30%	**40%**
Nuuchahnulth (Nootka) ET 12.6	20%	20%	**60%**
Umatilla ET 13.3	30%	30%	**40%**
Tenino ET 13.3	20%	30%	**50%**
Seri ET 18.3	25%	25%	**50%**
HUNTER-FISHER (ET 9.5–10.3)	*Hunt*	*Gather*	*Fish*
Iglulingmiut ET 9.5	**50%**	0	50%
Chipewyan ET 10.3	**60%**	0	40%
HUNTER-FISHER-GATHERER (ET 8.9–12.7)	*Hunt*	*Gather*	*Fish*
Yukaghir ET 8.9	**50%**	10%	40%

	Hunt	Gather	Fish
Ona Selk'nam ET 9.0	**70%**	10%	20%
Ojibwa ET 10.7	**40%**	30%	30%
Tanana ET 10.9	**70%**	10%	20%
Plains Cree ET 11.5	**60%**	20%	20%
Micmac ET 12.7	**50%**	10%	40%

HUNTER-GATHERER-FISHER **(ET 10.7–21.2)**	*Hunt*	*Gather*	*Fish*
Ojibwa ET 10.7	**40%**	30%	30%
Assiniboin ET 11.7	**70%**	20%	10%
Wind River Shoshone ET 12.0	**50%**	30%	20%
Kariera ET 18.0	**50%**	30%	20%
Aeta ET 21.2	**60%**	35%	5%

HUNTER-GATHERER (ET 11.3–16.5)	*Hunt*	*Gather*	*Fish*
Sarsi ET 11.3	**80%**	20%	0
Cheyenne ET 13.3	**80%**	20%	0
Kiowa-Apache ET 14.3	**80%**	20%	0
Comanche ET 14.4	**90%**	10%	0
Aweikoma ET 16.5	**60%**	40%	0

GATHERER-HUNTER-FISHER **(ET 11.7–23.7)**	*Hunt*	*Gather*	*Fish*
Ute (Uintah) ET 11.7	35%	**40%**	25%
Tubatulabal ET 12.9	30%	**50%**	20%
W. Mono ET 13.4	40%	**50%**	10%
Sierra Miwok ET 14.8	30%	**60%**	10%
Sirionoa ET 20.6	25%	**70%**	5%
Chenchua ET 20.8	10%	**85%**	5%
Tiwi ET 22.6	30%	**50%**	20%
Semanga ET 23.7	35%	**50%**	15%

GATHERER-FISHER-HUNTER (ET 12.7–24.4)	*Hunt*	*Gather*	*Fish*
Coast Yuki ET 12.7	20%	**40%**	**40%**
Kuyuidokad (Lake Paiute) ET 13.3	20%	**50%**	30%
Luiseno ET 15.1	20%	**60%**	20%
Nukak ET 21.7	11%	**76%**	13%
Onge (Andamanese) ET 24.4	20%	**40%**	**40%**

GATHERER-HUNTER (ET 14.0–19.3)	*Hunt*	*Gather*	*Fish*
Kaibab (S. Paiute) ET 14.0	30%	**70%**	0
Kade G/wi ET 14.8	20%	**80%**	0
Moapa ET 15.2	40%	**60%**	0
Hadza ET 17.7	35%	**65%**	0
Ju/'hoansi (Dobe) ET 18.8	20%	**80%**	0
G/wi ET 19.3	15%	**85%**	0

The remarkable variety of diets shown here reflects not just changing latitude, temperature ranges, environment and resources, but also the range of cultural adaptions demanded by that variety (all those regimes have inevitably been further refined by natural selection). The blanket term 'hunter-gatherer', although a convenient shorthand, is a quite inadequate description of these cultures, since the hunting, fishing and gathering ratios vary so markedly. That said, all the 126 regimes listed by Professor Kelly include some meat or fish: none are wholly vegetarian.

APPENDIX 2: DISEASES OF CIVILISATION: OSTEOLOGICAL EVIDENCE FROM BRITISH CEMETERY EXCAVATIONS

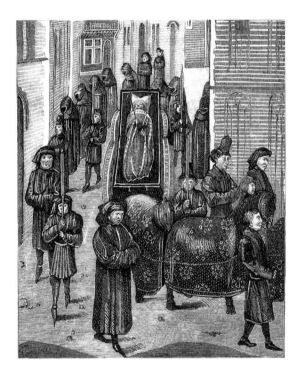

Fourteenth century funerary procession.

This summary table is based on the work of Professor Charlotte Roberts and Professor Margaret Cox (2003) and their palaeopathological study of 34,797 skeletons from 311 cemetery sites. They identified osteological evidence for illness related to, for example, dental, joint, metabolic and infectious diseases. This work enabled them to draw up a history of health and disease in Britain over many millennia, long before any formal written public health records were made (see also Hassett 2017). Their work provides unequivocal evidence of an alarming range of diseases and conditions that only appear *after* the advent of farming and urbanisation: the majority of the diseases catalogued here in **bold** were noticeably absent in the many millennia before civilisation arrived.

Period	Date range	Culture and diseases	Evidence
Palaeolithic/Mesolithic	10,500/8000–4000 BC	Hunter-gatherer style regimes	Some evidence of dental caries, dental defects, tooth loss; joint disease. No evidence of infections.
Neolithic	4000–2500 BC	Diseases of agrarianism	Increase in dental caries, dental defects, tooth loss; metabolic and joint disease; trauma. First evidence of **tumours, anaemia, diffuse idiopathic skeletal hyperostosis (DISH), osteoporosis, osteochondritis dissecans.** First evidence of infections such as **periostitis, osteitis, periostitis of sinuses, ribs and skull (possible meningitis).**
Later Prehistoric	2600 BC–AD 100	Bronze and Iron Age tribal cultures	Increase in dental caries, dental defects, tooth loss; anaemia; metabolic and joint disease; trauma. First evidence of **spondylosis; particular tumours (e.g. ostemas), osteomyelitis, os acromiale; spina bifida occulta.** New congenital and neoplastic (tumour) problems (e.g. **benign osteochondroma soft-tissue induced meningioma**); circulatory conditions such as **Scheuermann's and Perthes' disease.**
Roman	AD 50–AD 500	Diseases of early urbanisation	Increase in dental caries, dental defects, tooth loss; infections; trauma; anaemia; joint disease; os acromiale; sinusitis; rib periostitis; DISH, osteoporosis. First evidence of diet-related diseases such as **scurvy, rickets, osteomalacia.** First evidence of infections such as **leprosy, tuberculosis** (perhaps from infected cattle?), **osteitis; septic arthritis; poliomyelitis.** First evidence of new joint diseases such as **Reiter's syndrome; gout; ankylosing spondylitis; rheumatoid arthritis; psoriatic arthritis.**

Saxon	AD 500–AD 1000	Initially non-urbanised tribal society	Perhaps significantly for this study, there was a *decline* in dental disease, rates of anaemia, scurvy, rickets and osteoporosis, accompanied by an increase in average stature for males and females (to 1.72 m and 1.61 m respectively). As small towns developed later in this period there was an increase in infectious diseases (but no new ones), neoplastic and congenital disease.
Medieval	AD 1050–AD 1550	Growth of towns supplied by surplus from rural estates	Increase in dental, congenital, neoplastic and metabolic diseases; DISH; Paget's disease, osteoporosis; gall stones. Clear evidence for different disease profiles related to socio-economic status. First evidence of **bubonic plague** and **venereal syphilis**.
Early Modern	AD 1550–AD 1750		The rise and fall of urban diseases in the succeeding centuries can be traced partially through the study of human skeletal remains and increasingly through documented sources: for the 17th and 18th centuries the following entries were added to the contemporary death certificates: **plague, cholera, smallpox, measles, whooping cough, diphtheria, scarlet fever, typhus, dropsy, liver disease, asthma, pulmonary tuberculosis** and **various fevers.**

Source: Roberts and Cox 2003, chs. 2–6.

Postscript: our modern era

The list below is a reminder of the top ten killers in our modern age, all of which seem to have been rare or non-existent in 'uncivilised' societies. Is this because we are now living longer, and are thus prone to these conditions later in life? Such a solution has been suggested for the increased prevalence of fractures and osteoarthritis suffered by modern women in Athens, who now outlive many of their menfolk, a significant reversal of the situation represented by a study of a large cemetery site from the ancient Hellenistic town of Demetrias, founded in c.293 BC (Vanna 2007, 124–130). But is it acceptable to pass off our top ten killers (coronary heart disease, stroke/cerebrovascular disease, trachea/bronchus/lung cancer, lower respiratory infections, chronic obstructive pulmonary disease, Alzheimer's/dementia, colon/rectum cancers, diabetes, breast cancer, stomach cancer) just as 'diseases of old age', or might they relate more directly to our modern urban culture, rather than just increasing longevity?

APPENDIX 3: HUNTING, SPORT AND A GENDER AGENDA

Attributes such as extreme physical aggression, throwing projectiles, running and teamworking, which evolved primarily to support the particular but once necessary rigours of Palaeolithic hunting, were subsequently subsumed into inter-tribal combat and, as civilisations developed, all-out warfare. Those basic drives and dispositions are therefore deeply embedded in our genome, but are best expressed in more peaceful times through the medium of sport, especially team sports – a modern proxy for hunting.

Recent research in the United States (e.g. Deaner et al. 2012) has discussed such concepts, and also the related question of whether women are less disposed (not less able) to undertake team sports than men. That question is of particular relevance in the United States since the enactment of a federal law (Title IX) in 1972 prohibited sexual discrimination in educational opportunities, including sports. This resulted in the creation of substantially more opportunities and incentives for female athletes: in 1972, for example, females comprised 7% of high school athletes, but by 2010 that figure had rocketed to 42%. This profound change has been interpreted as indicating that the disposition of females towards sport is intrinsically equal to that of males, and that the opportunities facilitated by Title IX simply allowed females to better express their interest. But is that actually the case? After all, there is pronounced sexual dimorphism in musculature, strength and speed between men and women, and there is a large body of evidence, from sources ancient and modern, to support the case that males have a greater interest in sport than females. The surge in female sports participation in the United States since 1972 is certainly remarkable, but might the statistics be telling a more nuanced (but equally interesting) story?

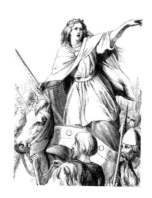

Boudicca, the warrior queen who led the fight against
Roman invaders in the first century AD.

Three studies were set up to consider this issue (Deaner et al. 2012, summarised below). Significantly, the participation in sport recorded for males and females was broken down into (a) team sports, (b) individual sports and (c) general exercise. This proved a significant distinction: substantial differences in the percentages of participation recorded in each category highlight differences, not in aptitude, but in attitude.

Study 1: Based on the American Time Use Survey (ATUS) of a sample of US residents aged 15 years and older. It was conducted from 2003 to 2010 and included responses from 112,000 individuals. Male participation rates were significantly higher than female rates for team sports and substantially higher for individual sports, contrasting with a range of 33% among females aged 15 to 19 but 29% for other age groups. However, for general exercise (e.g. aerobics, running, walking, yoga) female participation was actually greater.

	Team sport	**Individual sport**	**Exercise**
Male	80%	c. 70%	49%
Female	20%	29–33%	51%

Study 2: Observations of unorganised sports and exercise regimes at public parks in Grand Rapids, Michigan; State College, Pennsylvania; Tallahassee, Florida; and New Paltz, New York. Studies were undertaken in summer and autumn 2011 and spring 2012, documenting 2,879 participants. Again, the sex difference was significantly greater for team sports than individual sports, but noticeably less for exercise.

	Team sport	**Individual sport**	**Exercise**
Male	90%	81%	63%
Female	10%	19%	37%

Study 3: Survey of undergraduate participation in sport in colleges and universities, based on recorded registrations in 34 institutions in 2010 and 2011. Sports recorded by these 18- to 24-year-olds are played 'for fun', not at the more prestigious and demanding intercollegiate level. As such, they provide an indicator of intrinsic motivation to participate. Females accounted for 26% of total registrations across all institutions and sports: the median value was 28%, but there was no institution where female registration reached more than 43%.

	Team sport	Individual sport
Male	74%	69%
Female	26%	31%

Summary: Working with the three sub-categories, it seems that team sports (our hunting proxy) proved to be male dominated, whereas individual sports were less so, and general exercise not at all. Such a significant modern societal distinction seems to owe as much to our deep evolutionary past as to modern cultural preferences. Arguably, the men were from Mars (still), whereas the women were demonstrating a greater adaptability to 21st-century life.

APPENDIX 4: HOW GREEN IS YOUR CITY?

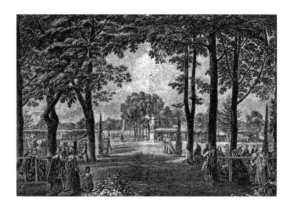

Tiergarten, Berlin in 1772.

How much greenspace do we have in our towns? UK town planners characterise greenspaces in their Planning Policy Guidance (PPG) notes with these broadly functionalist headings:[1]

1. Parks and gardens, including urban parks and formal gardens.

2. Natural and semi-natural urban greenspaces, including woodlands, wetlands and wastelands.

3. Green corridors, including river and canal banks.

4. Outdoor sports facilities, including tennis courts and school playing fields.

5. Amenity greenspace, including informal recreation spaces in and around housing.

6. Provision for children and teenagers, including play areas and skateboard parks.

7. Allotments, community gardens and city farms.

8. Civic spaces, including market squares and other hard-surfaced areas.

9. Cemeteries and churchyards.

10. Accessible countryside in urban fringe areas.

---

1   An additional facility, non-urban greenspace (e.g. national parks), exists beyond our urban administrative boundaries, and therefore often beyond the legal remit of the city authority.

Urban greenspace is beneficial in providing opportunities for physical activity and social interaction as well as for the promotion of biodiversity. The level of engagement with nature varies considerably (for the most intensive versions, see (7) and (8) below). The headings below have been modified from those in the list above to reflect the ownership of the land (and thus where the prime responsibility for their maintenance and development lies), and how various greenspaces are currently used.

1. Public recreational urban greenspace: extensive lands, large parks or heaths, e.g. Hampstead Heath/Hyde Park; also bowling greens and sports fields maintained by the urban authority or state organisations such as royal parks. (PPG17: natural and semi-natural urban greenspaces; also outdoor sports facilities, parks and gardens)

2. Non-local-authority recreational urban greenspace: e.g. privately maintained sports fields, golf courses. (PPG17: outdoor sports facilities)

3. Public linear urban greenspace/bluespace: includes routes alongside rivers (e.g. Thames Path) and canals (e.g. Regents Canal) or over disused railway lines (e.g. Hornsey). There are now some 40 designated 'greenways' in the London area, designed to accommodate pedestrians and cyclists in a largely traffic-free environment. The routes run through parks, alongside waterways or on the quieter residential streets. By 2012, this network extended for 375 km, and there are ambitious plans to extend the total to 1,900 km. (PPG17: green corridors)

4. Civic space: market squares or pedestrianised areas designed for social focus and interaction. (PPG17: civic spaces)

5. Neighbourhood urban greenspace: landscaped squares, small parks, greens, pavement, trees, flowerbeds, planters, etc. Features maintained by urban authority. (PPG17: amenity greenspace)

6. Devotional urban greenspace: e.g. publicly accessible cemeteries and churchyards. (PPG17: cemeteries and churchyards)

7. Participatory urban greenspace: e.g. allotments, community gardens, community orchards, community meadows, therapeutic gardens, urban farms. Often maintained by community effort, often by those without private gardens, but sometimes owned by an urban authority.

8. Private urban greenspace: e.g. residential gardens, patios, roof gardens.

9. Enclosed linear urban greenspace: formed by cuttings/embankments of e.g. railway network – important wildlife corridors and havens of biodiversity. Maintained by transport companies but fenced off from the public.

REFERENCES AND FURTHER READING

Abdallah, A., Steuer, N., Marks, N. and Page, N. (2008) *Well-Being Evaluation Tools: A Research and Development Project for the Big Lottery Fund Final Report*. London: New Economics Foundation.

Abercrombie, P. (1944) *Greater London Plan*. London: University of London Press.

Aiello, L. and Wheeler, P. (1995) 'The expensive-tissue hypothesis: the brain and the digestive system in human and primate evolution', *Current Anthropology* 36, 199–221.

Aked, J., Marks, N., Cordon, C. and Thompson, S. (2009) *Five Ways to Wellbeing: A Report Presented to the Foresight Project on Communicating the Evidence Base for Improving People's Well-Being*. London: New Economics Foundation.

Alexander, C. (1965) 'A city is not a tree', *Architectural Forum* 122(1), 58–62.

Allan, C. B. and Lutz, W. (1967) *Life Without Bread: How a Low-Carbohydrate Diet Can Save Your Life* [Leben Ohne Brot]. New York: McGraw-Hill Education.

American Diabetes Association (2016) 'Obesity management for the treatment of type 2 diabetes', *Diabetes Care* 39 (Suppl. 1), S47–S51. Available at: http://dx.doi.org/10.2337/dc16-S009.

Anderson, D. (2016) 'Story of cities #future: what will our growing megacities really look like?' *The Guardian* (26 May). Available at: https://www.theguardian.com/cities/2016/may/26/story-cities-future-growing-megacities-waste-floating-smart.

Andrews, P. (2015) *An Ape's View of Human Evolution*. Cambridge: Cambridge University Press.

Arab, L. and Ang, A. (2015) 'A cross sectional study of the association between walnut consumption and cognitive function among adult US populations represented in NHANES', *Journal of Nutrition, Health and Aging* 19(3), 284–290. Available at: http://link.springer.com/article/10.1007/s12603-014-0569-2.

Armelagos, G. (1990) 'Disease in prehistoric populations in transition', in A. Swedlund and G. Armelagos (eds), *Disease in Populations in Transition: Anthropological and Epidemiological Perspective*. South Hadley, MA: Bergin and Garvey, pp. 124–142.

Ashmore, T., Fernandez, B., Branco-Price, C., West, J., Cowburn, A., Heather, L., Griffin, J., Johnson, R., Feelisch, M. and Murray, A. (2014a) 'Dietary nitrate increases arginine availability and protects mitochondrial complex I and energetics in the hypoxic rat heart', *Journal of Physiology* 592, 4715–4731.

Ashmore, T., Fernandez, B., Evans, C., Huang, Y., Branco-Price, C., Griffin, J., Johnson, R., Feelisch, M. and Murray, A. (2014b) 'Suppression of erythropoiesis by dietary nitrate', *Journal of the Federation of American Societies for Experimental Biology* 29(3), 1102–1112.

Aspinall, P., Marvos, P., Coyne, R. and Roe, J. (2013) 'The urban brain: analysing outdoor physical activity with mobile EEG', *British Journal of Sports Medicine* 49(4), 272–276. DOI: 10.1136/bjsports-2012-091877

Atkins, R. (1972) *Dr Atkins' Diet Revolution: The High Calorie Way to Stay Thin Forever*. New York: Bantam Doubleday Dell Publishing Group.

Atkins, R. (2002) *Dr Atkins' New Diet Revolution*. London: Vermilion.

Audette, R. (1995) *NeanderThin: Eat Like a Caveman to Achieve a Lean, Strong, Healthy Body*. New York: St Martin's Press.

Baker, J. and Brookes, S. (2013) *Beyond the Burghal Hidage: Anglo-Saxon Civil Defence in the Viking Age*. Leiden and Boston, MA: Brill.

Ball, L. J. and Birge, S. J. (2002) 'Prevention of brain aging and dementia', *Clinics in Geriatric Medicine* 18(3), 485–503.

Bannan, N. (ed.) (2012a) *Music, Language, and Human Evolution*. Oxford: Oxford University Press.

Bannan, N. (2012b) 'Music, language, and human evolution', in N. Bannan (ed.), *Music, Language, and Human Evolution*. Oxford: Oxford University Press, pp. 3–27.

Banting, W. (1863) *Letters on Corpulence*. London: Harrison & Sons.

Barkow, J., Cosmides, L. and Tooby, J. (1992) *The Adapted Mind: Evolutionary Psychology and the Generation of Culture*. Oxford: Oxford University Press.

Barnard, A. (2011) *Social Anthropology and Human Origins*. Cambridge: Cambridge University Press.

Barnard, A. (2016) *Language in Prehistory*. Cambridge: Cambridge University Press.

Barrett, L., Dunbar, R. and Lycett, J. (2002) *Human Evolutionary Psychology*. London: Palgrave.

Barrett, P., Zhang, Y., Moffat, J. and Kobbacy, K. (2013) 'A holistic, multi-level analysis identifying the impact of classroom design on pupil's learning', *Building and Environment* 59, 678–689.

Barton, J. and Pretty, J. (2010) 'What is the best dose of nature and green exercise for improving mental health? A multi-study analysis', *Environmental Science and Technology* 44(10), 3947–3955.

BBC (2013) '*Call of Duty* dominates 2012 entertainment sales beating music and film' (13 March). Available at: http://www.bbc.co.uk/news/technology-21769023.

Bellamy, E. (1888) *Looking Backward, 2000–1887*. Boston, MA: Ticknor and Co.

Berger, A. (2007) *Drosscape: Wasting Land in Urban America*. Princeton, NJ: Princeton Architectural Press.

Berger, L., Hawks, J., de Ruiter, D. J., Churchill, S. E., Schmid, P., Delezeneet, L. K. et al. (2015) '*Homo naledi*, a new species of the genus *Homo* from the Dinaledi Chamber, South Africa', *eLife* 4: e09560. Available at: https://elifesciences.org/content/4/e09560.

Berman, M. (2000) *Wandering God: A Study in Nomadic Spirituality*. Albany, NY: State University of New York Press.

Biddle, J. H. and Ekkekakis, P. (2005) 'Physically active lifestyles and wellbeing', in F. Huppert, N. Baylis and B. Keveme (eds), *The Science of Well-Being*. Oxford: Oxford University Press, pp. 140–168.

Biddle, M. (1970) 'Excavations at Winchester, 1969', *Antiquaries Journal* 50: 277–326.

Blacking, J. (1973) *How Musical is Man?* Seattle, WA: University of Washington Press.

Blackley, C. (1873) *Experimental Researches in the Cause and Nature of Catarrhus Aestivus*. London: Baillière, Tindall & Cox.

Blane, D. (2006) 'The life course, the social gradient and health', in M. G. Marmot and R. G. Wilkinson (eds), *Social Determinants of Health*. Oxford: Oxford University Press, pp. 54–77.

Bloom, H. (2000) *Global Brain: The Evolution of Mass Mind from the Big Bang to the 21st Century*. Toronto: John Wiley & Sons.

Blumenthal, J. A., Babyak, M. A., Moore, K. A., Craighead, W. E., Herman, S., Khatri, P., Waugh, R., Napolitano, M. A., Forman, L. M., Appelbaum, M., Doraiswamy, P. M. and Krishnan, K. R. (1999) 'Effects of exercise training on older patients with major depression', *Archives of Internal Medicine* 159, 2349–2356.

Borland, S. (2014) 'Slap a sugar tax on fizzy drinks and junk food: shock call by chief medical officer', *Daily Mail* (4 March). Available at: http://www.dailymail.co.uk/health/article-2573368/Slap-sugar-tax-fizzy-drinks-junk-food-Shock-call-chief-medical-officer.html.

Borst, H., Miedema, H., de Vries, A., Graham, J. and van Dongen, J. (2008) 'Relationships between street characteristics and perceived attractiveness for walking reported by elderly people', *Journal of Environmental Psychology* 28(4), 353–361. DOI: 10.1016/j.jenvp.2008.02.010

Bowman, K. (2015) *Don't Just Sit There*. Sequim, WA: Propriometric Press.

Bramble, D. and Lieberman, D. (2004) 'Endurance running and the evolution of Homo', *Nature* 432, 345–352. DOI: 10.1038/nature03052

Brooke, C. and Keir, G. (1975) *London 800–1216: The Shaping of a City*. London: Martin Secker & Warburg.

Brothwell, D. and Brothwell, P. (1998) *Food in Antiquity: A Survey of the Diet of Early Peoples*. Baltimore, MD: Johns Hopkins University Press.

Brown, S. (2000) 'The "musilanguage" model of music evolution', in N. Wallin, B. Merker and S. Brown (eds), *The Origins of Music*. Cambridge: MIT Press, pp. 271–301.

Brunner, E. and Marmot, M. (2006) 'Social organisation, stress and health', in M. Marmot and R. J. Wilkinson (eds), *Social Determinants of Health*. Oxford: Oxford University Press, pp. 6–30.

Bryant, V. (1979) 'I put myself on a caveman diet permanently', *Prevention* (Sept), 128–137.

Bryant, V. (1995) 'The Palaeolithic health club', *1995 Yearbook of Science and the Future*. Chicago, IL: Encyclopedia Britannica, pp. 114–133.

Burkitt, D., Walker, A. and Palmer, N. (1974) 'Dietary fiber and disease', *JAMA* 229, 1068–1074.

Calleau, J. (2005) 'The benefits of volunteers attending Cherry Tree Nursery', *Growth Point –Journal of Social and Therapeutic Horticulture* 101, 20–22.

Campbell, C. and Campbell, T. (2005) *The China Study*. Dallas, TX: BenBella Books.

Campbell, S. (2013) Keynote address at the North of England Education conference: Mind, Brain, Community: Inspiring Learners, Strengthening Resilience, 16 January, Sheffield Hallam University.

Cavill, N. and Rutter, H. (2013) *Healthy People, Healthy Places Briefing: Obesity and the Environment: Regulating the Growth of Fast Food Outlets*. London: Public Health England.

Cecil, C., Viding, E., Barker, E., Guiney, J. and McCrory, J. (2014) 'Double disadvantage: the influence of childhood maltreatment and community violence exposure on adolescent mental health', *Journal of Child Psychology and Psychiatry* 55(7), 839–848. DOI: 10.1111/jcpp.12213

Chagnon, N. (1997) *The Yanomamo* (Case Studies in Cultural Anthropology). Orlando, FL: Harcourt Brace.

Chaitow, L. (1987) *Stone Age Diet: The Natural Way to Eat*. London: Optima.

Childe, V. G. (1950) 'The urban revolution', *Town Planning Review* 21(1), 3–17.

Choi, J., Beltran, L. and Kim, H. (2012) 'Impacts of indoor daylight environments on patient average length of stay in a healthcare facility', *Building and Environment* 50, 65–75.

Cleave, T. (1974) *The Saccharine Disease*. Oxford: Butterworth-Heinemann.

Clegg, M. (2012) 'The Evolution of the vocal tract', in R. Bannan (ed.), *Music, Language, and Human Evolution*. Oxford: Oxford University Press, pp. 58–80.

Cohen, D. (2016) 'The boat club is a sanctuary, where young people can be fed, be safe … be children', *Evening Standard* (4 March), p. 8.

Cohen, M. N. (2012) 'History, diet, and hunter-gatherers', in K. F. Kiple and C. O. Kriemhild (eds), *The Cambridge World History of Food*. Cambridge: Cambridge University Press, pp. 63–71.

CoL (Corporation of London) (1944) *Reconstruction in the City of London: Preliminary Draft Proposals for Post-War Reconstruction in the City of London*. London: B.T. Batsford.

Conard, N. J. (2003) 'Palaeolithic ivory sculptures from southwestern Germany and the origins of figurative art', *Nature* 426, 830–832.

Congress for New Urbanism (n.d.) The Charter of the New Urbanism. Available at: https://www.cnu.org/who-we-are/charter-new-urbanism.

Cordain, L. (2012 [2002]) *The Paleo Diet: Lose Weight and Get Healthy by Eating the Food You Were Designed to Eat*. New York: Wiley.

Cordain, L., Eaton, S. B., Sebastian, A., Mann, N., Lindeberg, S., Watkins, B., O'Keefe, J. and Brand Miller, J. (2005) 'Origins and evolution of the Western diet: health implications for the 21st century', *American Journal of Clinical Nutrition* 81, 341–354.

Cordain, L., Gotshall, R., Eaton, S. B. and Eaton, S. B. III (1998) 'Physical activity, energy expenditure and fitness: an evolutionary perspective', *International Journal of Sports Medicine* 19, 328–335.

Cordain, L., Miller, J. B. and Eaton, S. B. (2000) 'Plant-animal subsistence ratios and macronutrient energy estimations in worldwide hunter-gatherer diets', *American Journal of Clinical Nutrition* 71, 682–692.

Coward, F., Horsfield, R., Pope, M. and Wenban-Smith, F. (eds) (2015) *Settlement, Society and Cognition in Human Evolution*. Cambridge: Cambridge University Press.

Cranz, G. (1982) *The Politics of Park Design: A History of Urban Parks in America*. Cambridge, MA: MIT Press.

Cronon, W. (1995) 'The trouble with wilderness', in W. Cronon (ed.), *Uncommon Ground: Rethinking the Human Place in Nature*. New York: W.W. Norton, pp. 69–90.

Cummings, V., Jordan, P. and Zvelebil, M. (2014) *The Oxford Handbook of the Archaeology and Anthropology of Hunter-Gatherers*. Oxford: Oxford University Press.

Cupchik, W. and Atcheson, D. J. (1983) 'Shoplifting: an occasional crime of the moral majority', *Journal of the American Academy of Psychiatry and the Law* 11(4): 343–354.

d'Errico, F. (2003) 'Neanderthal extinction and the millennial scale climatic variability of OIS 3', *Quaternary Science Reviews* 22, 769–788.

Dannenberg, A., Frumkin, H. and Jackson, R. J. (2011) *Making Healthy Places: A Built Environment for Health, Well-Being, and Sustainability*. Washington, DC: Island Press.

Darwin, C. (1859) *On the Origin of Species by Means of Natural Selection, Or the Preservation of Favoured Races in the Struggle for Life*. London: John Murray.

Darwin, C. (1871) *The Descent of Man and Selection in Relation to Sex*. London: John Murray.

Darwin, E. (1794) *Zoonomia; or, The Laws of Organic Life*. London: J. Johnson.

Dawkins, R. (1976) *The Selfish Gene*. Oxford: Oxford University Press.

de Busk, R. (2010) 'The role of nutritional genomics in developing an optimal diet for humans', *Nutrition in Clinical Practice* 25, 627–633.

de Vany, A. (2011) *The New Evolution Diet: What Our Palaeolithic Ancestors Can Teach Us About Weight Loss, Fitness and Ageing*. New York: Rodale Books.

Deaner, R. O., Geary, D. C., Puts, D. A., Ham, S. A., Kruger, J., Fles, E. et al. (2012) 'A sex difference in the predisposition for physical competition: males play sports much more than females even in the contemporary US', *PLoS ONE* 7(11): e49168. DOI: 10.1371/journal.pone.0049168

DEFRA (2012) *Family Food 2012*. London: Department for Environment, Food and Rural Affairs.

DEFRA (2015) *Improving Air Quality in the UK: Tackling Nitrogen Dioxide in Our Towns and Cities. UK Overview Document* (December). London: Department for Environment, Food and Rural Affairs.

Denbow, J. (1984) 'Prehistoric herders and foragers of the Kalahari: the evidence of 1,500 years of interaction', in C. Schrire (ed.), *Past and Present in Hunter-Gatherer Studies*. New York: Academic Press, pp. 175–193.

Department for Communities and Local Government (2006) Planning Policy Guidance 17: Planning for Open Space, Sport and Recreation (PPG17).

Derr, M. (2011) *How the Dog Became the Dog: From Wolves to Our Best Friends*. New York: Penguin.

Digard, L., von Sponek, A. G. and Liebling, A. (2007) 'All Together Now: the therapeutic potential of a prison-based music programme', *Prison Service Journal* 170, 3–14.

DiNicolantonio, J. and Lucan, S. C. (2014) 'Cardiac risk factors and prevention. The wrong white crystals: not salt but sugar as aetiological in hypertension and cardiometabolic disease', *Open Heart* 2014(1): e000167. DOI: 10.1136/openhrt-2014-000167

DoH (2012) *National Diet and Nutrition Survey: Headline Results from Years 1, 2 and 3 (Combined) of the Rolling Programme (2008/09–2010/11)*. London: Department of Health. Available at: https://www.gov.uk/government/statistics/national-diet-and-nutrition-survey-headline-results-from-years-1-2-and-3-combined-of-the-rolling-programme-200809-201011.

DoH (2014) *Results of the National Diet and Nutrition Survey (NDNS) Rolling Programme for 2008 and 2009 to 2011 and 2012*. London: Department of Health. Available at: https://www.gov.uk/government/statistics/national-diet-and-nutrition-survey-results-from-years-1-to-4-combined-of-the-rolling-programme-for-2008-and-2009-to-2011-and-2012.

Doyle, A. C. (2001 [1887]) *A Study in Scarlet*. London: Penguin.

Dunbar, R. (1998) 'Theory of mind and the evolution of language', in R. Hurford, M. Studdert-Kennedy and C. Knight (eds), *Approaches to the Evolution of Language*. Cambridge: Cambridge University Press, pp. 92–110.

Dunbar, R. (2004a) *The Human Story*. London: Faber & Faber.

Dunbar, R. (2004b) 'Language, music and laughter in evolutionary perspective', in D. Oller and U. Griebel (eds), *Evolution of Communication Systems*. Cambridge, MA: MIT Press, pp. 257–274.

Dunbar, R. (2012) 'On the evolutionary function of song and dance', in R. Bannan (ed.), *Music, Language, and Human Evolution*. Oxford: Oxford University Press, pp. 201–214.

Dunbar, R. (2014) *Human Evolution*. Pelican: London.

Dunbar, R. and Barrett, L. (eds) (2007) *Oxford Handbook of Evolutionary Psychology*. Oxford: Oxford University Press.

Dunbar, R., Gamble, C. and Gowlett, J. (eds) (2010) *Social Brain, Distributed Mind* (Proceedings of the British Academy). Oxford: Oxford University Press.

Dunbar, R., Gamble, C. and Gowlett, J. (eds) (2014) *Lucy to Language: The Benchmark Papers*. Oxford: Oxford University Press.

Duncan, D. F. (1985) 'The Peckham Experiment: a pioneering exploration of wellness', *Health Values* 9(5), 40–43.

Easterlin, R. A. (1974) 'Does economic growth improve the human lot?' in P. David and M. Reder (eds), *Nations and Households in Economic Growth: Essays in Honor of Moses Abramovitz*. New York: Academic Press, pp. 89–125.

Eaton, S. B. and Konner, M. (1985) 'Palaeolithic nutrition: a consideration of its nature and current implications', *New England Journal of Medicine* 312(5), 283–289.

Eaton, S. B., Shostak, M. and Konner, M. (1985) *The Palaeolithic Prescription: A Program of Diet and Exercise and a Design for Living*. New York: Harper and Row.

Eaton, S. B., Shostak, M. and Konner, M. (1989) *Stone Age Health Programme: Diet and Exercise as Nature Intended*. London: Angus and Robertson.

Edgeworth, M., Richter, D., Waters, C., Haff, P., Neal, C. and Price, S. (2015) 'Diachronous beginnings of the Anthropocene: the lower bounding surface of anthropogenic deposits', *Anthropocene Review* 2, 33–58.

Elzeyadi, I. (2011) 'Daylighting-bias and biophilia: quantifying the impacts of daylight on occupants health', in *Thought and Leadership in Green Buildings Research: Greenbuild 2011 Proceedings*. Washington, DC: USGBC Press.

Enard, W., Przeworski, M., Fisher, S., Lai, C., Wiebe, V., Kitano, T., Monaco, A. and Pääbo, S. (2002) 'Molecular evolution of FOXP2, a gene involved in speech and language', *Nature* 418, 869–872. DOI: 10.1038/nature01025

Esliger, D., Trembaly, M., Copeland, J., Barnes, J., Huntingdon, G. and Bassett, D. (2010) 'Physical activity profile of Old Order Amish, Mennonite and contemporary children', *Medicine and Science in Sports and Exercise* 42, 296–303. DOI: 10.1249/MSS.0b013e3181b3afd2

Ewing, C., MacDonald, P., Taylor, M. and Bowers, M. (2007) 'Equine-facilitated learning for youths with severe emotional disorders: a quantitative and qualitative study', *Child Youth Care Forum* 36, 59–72.

Fediuk, K. (2000) Vitamin C in the Inuit diet: past and present. MA thesis, School of Dietetics and Human Nutrition, McGill University, Montreal.

Felson, M. (2006) *Crime and Nature*. Thousand Oaks, CA: Sage.

Foley, R. (2012) 'Music and mosaics: the evolution of human abilities', in N. Bannan (ed.), *Music, Language, and Human Evolution*. Oxford: Oxford University Press, pp. 31–57.

Frumkin, H. (2001) 'Beyond toxicity: human health and the natural environment', *American Journal of Preventive Medicine* 20(3), 234–240.

Fuller, D., Kingwell-Banham, E., Lucas, L., Murphy, C. and Stevens, C. (2015) 'Comparing pathways to agriculture', *Archaeology International* 18, 61–66.

Gardner, B. and Wardle, J. (2012) 'The role of health behaviour', in D. French, K. Vedhara, A. Kaptein and J. Weinman (eds), *Health Psychology* (2nd edn). Oxford: Blackwell, pp. 13–32.

Garmonsway, G. (ed.) (1972) *The Anglo Saxon Chronicle*. London: J. M. Dent & Sons.

Garreau, J. (1992) *Edge City: Life on the New Frontier*. Garden City, NY: Anchor Books.

Gerbault, P., Roffet-Salque, M., Evershed, R. and Thomas, M. (2013) 'How long have adult humans been consuming milk?' *International Union of Biochemistry and Molecular Biology* 65, 983–990.

Germonpré, M., Sablin, M., Stevens, R., Hedges, R., Hofreiter, M., Stiller, M. and Despres, V. (2009) 'Fossil dogs and wolves from Palaeolithic sites in Belgium, the Ukraine and Russia: osteometry, ancient DNA and stable isotopes', *Journal of Archaeological Science* 36, 473–490.

Gilliland, J., Rivet, D. and Fitzpatrick, S. (2012) *Healthy City/Active London: Evidence-Based Recommendations for Policies to Promote Walking and Biking*. London, ON: Middlesex–London Health Unit.

Gladwell, L. (2007) 'Gardening at the Berkshire adolescent unit at Wokingham hospital', *Growth Point – Journal of Social and Therapeutic Horticulture* 110, 4–8.

Gordon, R. (1984) 'The !Kung in the Kalahari Exchange: an ethnohistorical perspective', in C. Schrire (ed.), *Past and Present in Hunter-Gatherer Studies*. New York: Academic Press, pp. 195–224.

Gremillion, K. (2011) *Ancestral Appetites*. Cambridge: Cambridge University Press.

Grootveld, M., Ruiz-Rodado, V. and Silwood, C. (2014) 'Detection, monitoring and deleterious health effects of lipid oxidation products generated in culinary oils during thermal stressing episodes', *Inform, American Oil Chemists' Society* 25(10), 614–624.

Hamblin, J. (1997) 'Has the garden of Eden been located at last?' Available at: www.ldolphin.org./eden.

Hancock, T. (1993) 'The evolution, impact and significance of the health cities/health communities movement', *Journal of Public Health Policy* 14, 5–18.

Harari, Y. N. (2014) *Sapiens: A Brief History of Humankind*. London: Harvill Secker.

Hardy, K., Brand-Miller, J., Brown, K. D., Thomas, M. G. and Copeland, L. (2015) 'The importance of dietary carbohydrate in human evolution', *Quarterly Review of Biology* 90, 251–268.

Harris, E. E. (2014) *Ancestors in Our Genome: The New Science of Human Evolution*. Oxford: Oxford University Press.

Hart, C., Pilling, A. and Goodale, J. (1988) *The Tiwi of North Australia* (Case Studies in Cultural Anthropology). New York: Holt, Rinehart and Winston.

Hartmann, D. and Depro, B. (2006) 'Rethinking sports-based community crime prevention: a preliminary analysis of the relationship between midnight basketball and urban crime rates', *Journal of Sport and Social Issues* 30, 180–196.

Harwood, E. (2001) 'Lansbury', in E. Harwood and A. Powers (eds), *Festival of Britain* (Twentieth Century Architecture 5). London: Twentieth Century Society, pp. 139–154.

Harwood, E. and Powers, A. (eds) (2001) *Festival of Britain* (Twentieth Century Architecture 5). London: Twentieth Century Society.

Hassett, B. (2017) *Built on Bones: 15,000 Years of Urban Life and Death*. London: Bloomsbury Sigma.

Hassink, J. and van Dijk, M. (eds) (2006) *Farming for Health: Green-Care Farming Across Europe and the United States of America*. Dordrecht: Springer.

Healey, T. and Cote, S. (2001) *The Wellbeing of Nations: The Role of Human and Social Capital*. Paris: OECD.

Herbert, M. (1999) 'A city in good shape: town planning and public health', *Town Planning Review* 70(4), 433–453.

Herbert, M. (2005) 'Engineering, urbanism and the struggle for street design', *Journal for Urban Design* 10(1), 39–59.

Heschong Mahone Group (1999) Daylighting in Schools: An Investigation into the Relationship Between Daylighting and Human Performance. Available at: http://h-m-g.com/downloads/Daylighting/schoolc.pdf.

Heylighen, F. (2010) 'Evolutionary well-being: the Paleolithic model', *ECCO* (22 June). Available at: http://ecco.vub.ac.be/?q=node/127.

Heylighen, F. (2014) 'Evolutionary psychology', in A. C. Michalos (ed.), *Encyclopedia of Quality of Life and WellBeing Research*. Dordrecht: Springer, pp. 2058–2062.

Hill, D. (1969) 'The Burghal Hidage: the establishment of a text', *Medieval Archaeology* 13, 84–92.

Hine, R., Peacock, J. and Pretty, J. (2007) Evaluating the Impact of Environmental Volunteering on Behaviours and Attitudes to the Environment. Report for BTCV Cymru/ University of Essex.

Hine, R., Peacock, J. and Pretty, J. (2008) Care Farming in the UK: Education and Opportunities. Report for the National Care Farming Initiative (UK)/University of Essex. Available at: http://www.carefarminguk.org/sites/carefarminguk.org/files/UK%20 Care%20Farming%20Research%20Study.pdf.

Hollick, M. F. (2006) 'Resurrection of vitamin D deficiency and rickets', *Journal of Clinical Investigation* 116, 2062–2072.

Hooker, J. (1859) *The Botany of the Antarctic Voyage of H.M. Discovery Ships Erebus and Terror in the Years 1839–1843, Under the Command of Captain Sir James Clark Ross [Flora Antarctica]: Flora of Tasmania*, 2 vols. London: Reeve Brothers.

Howard, E. (1902 [1898]) *Garden Cities of Tomorrow* (2nd edn). London: S. Sonnenschein and Co.

HSCIC (2015) *Dental Disease and Damage in Children: England, Wales and Northern Ireland: Children's Dental Health Survey 2013: Report 2*. London: Health and Social Care Information Centre. Available at: http://content.digital.nhs.uk/catalogue/PUB17137/ CDHS2013-Report2-Dental-Disease.pdf.

Hu, F. B. and Willett, W. C. (2002) 'Optimal diets for prevention of coronary heart disease', *JAMA* 288(20), 2569–2578.

Hunt, J. D. (2000) *Greater Perfections: The Practice of Garden Theory*. Philadelphia, PA: University of Pennsylvania Press.

Hurford, R., Studdert-Kennedy, M. and Knight, C. (eds) (1998) *Approaches to the Evolution of Language*. Cambridge: Cambridge University Press.

Hutton, J. (1785) Abstract of a dissertation read in the Royal Society of Edinburgh, upon the seventh of March, and fourth of April, 1785, Concerning the System of the Earth, Its Duration, and Stability. Edinburgh.

Huxley, T. (1863) *Evidence as to Man's Place in Nature*. London: Williams & Norwood.

Hyppönen, E. and Boucher, B. (2010) 'Avoidance of vitamin D deficiency in pregnancy in the UK: the case for a unified approach in national policy', *British Journal of Nutrition* 104, 309–314.

Hyppönen, E. and Power, C. (2007) 'Hypovitaminosis D in British adults at age 45 y: a nationwide cohort study on dietary and lifestyle predictors', *American Journal of Clinical Nutrition* 85, 860–868.

Itan, Y., Bryson, B. and Thomas, M. G. (2010) 'Detecting gene duplications in the human lineage', *Annals of Human Genetics* 74, 555–565. DOI: 10.1111/j.1469-1809.2010.00609.x

Itan, Y., Powell, A., Beaumont, M., Burger, J. and Thomas, M. G. (2009) 'The origins of lactase persistence in Europe', *PLOS Computational Biology* 5: e1000491.

Johanson, D. and Edgar, B. (1996) *From Lucy to Language*. New York: Simon & Schuster.

Jones, E., Gonzalez-Fortes, G., Connell, S., Siska, V., Eriksson, A., Martiniano, R. et al. (2015) 'Upper Palaeolithic genomes reveal deep roots of modern Eurasians', *Nature Communications* 6: e8912. DOI: 10.1038/ncomms9912

Kahn, P., Friedman, B., Gill, B., Hagman, J., Severson, R., Freier, N., Feldman, N., Carrere, S. and Stolyar, A. (2008) 'A plasma display window? The shifting baseline problem in a technologically mediated natural world', *Journal of Environmental Psychology* 28(2), 192–199.

Katz, D. L. and Meller, S. (2014) 'Can we say what diet is best health?' *Annual Review of Public Health* 35, 86–103.

Katz, P. (1994) *The New Urbanism*. New York: McGraw-Hill.

Keene, D. and Harding, V. (eds) (1985) *A Survey of Documentary Sources for Property Holding in London Before the Great Fire*, Vol. 22. London: London Record Society.

Kelly, R. L. (2013) *The Lifeways of Hunter-Gatherers: The Foraging Spectrum*. Cambridge: Cambridge University Press.

Keys, A. (1971) 'Sucrose in the diet and coronary heart disease', *Atherosclerosis* 14, 193–202.

Keys, A. (1975) 'Coronary heart disease – the global picture', *Atherosclerosis* 22, 149–192.

Keys, A. (1980) *Seven Countries: A Multivariate Analysis of Death and Coronary Heart Disease*. Cambridge, MA: Harvard University Press.

Kinsella, B. (2011) *Tackling Knife Crime Together: A Review of Local Anti-Knife Crime Projects*. London: Home Office. Available at: https://www.gov.uk/government/publications/tackling-knife-crime-together-a-review-of-local-anti-knife-crime-projects.

Kiple, K. F. and Kriemhild, C. O. (eds) (2012) *The Cambridge World History of Food*. Cambridge: Cambridge University Press.

Klein, M. (1995) *The American Street Gang: Its Nature, Prevalence and Control*. New York: Oxford University Press.

Klein, M., Kerner, H.-J., Maxson, C. and Weitekamp, E. (2001) *The Eurogang Paradox: Street Gangs and Youth Groups in the US and Europe*. Dordrecht: Springer.

Klein, R. (2009) *The Human Career: Human Biological and Cultural Origins* (3rd edn). Chicago, IL: University of Chicago Press.

Knudsen, V. K., Matthiessen, J., Biltoft-Jensen, A., Sørensen, M. R., Groth, M. V., Trolle, E., Christensen, T. and Fag, S. (2014) 'Identifying dietary patterns and associated health-related lifestyle factors in the adult Danish population', *European Journal of Clinical Nutrition* 68, 736–740.

Kolbert, E. (2014) *The Sixth Extinction: An Unnatural History*. New York: Henry Holt.

Kompier, M., Mulders, H., Meijman, T., Boersma, M., Groen, G. and Bullinga, R. (1990) 'Absence behaviour, turnover and disability: a study among city bus drivers in the Netherlands', *Work and Stress* 4, 83–89.

Konner, M. and Eaton, S. B. (2010) 'Palaeolithic nutrition: 25 years later', *Nutrition in Clinical Practice* 25, 594–602.

Korpela, K., Salonen, A., Virta, L., Kekkonen, R. and de Vos, W. (2016) 'Association of early-life antibiotic use and protective effects of breastfeeding: role of the intestinal microbiota', *JAMA Pediatrics* 170(8), 750–757. DOI: 10.1001/jamapediatrics.2016.238

Kuo, F. E., Bacaicoa, M. and Sullivan, W. C. (1998) 'Transforming inner-city landscapes: trees, sense of safety, and preference', *Environment and Behaviour* 30, 28–59.

Kweon, B., Sullivan, W. C. and Wiley, A. R. (1998) 'Green common spaces and the social integration of inner-city older adults', *Environment and Behaviour* 30, 832–858.

Laden, G. and Wrangham, R. (2005) 'The rise of the hominids as an adaptive shift in fallback foods', *Journal of Human Evolution* 49, 482–492.

Lamarck, J. (1830) *Philosophie zoologique* (2nd edn), 2 vols. Paris: Germer Baillière. Available at: https://archive.org/details/philosophiezool02unkngoog.

Larsen, C. S. (1981) 'Skeletal and dental adaptions to the shift to agriculture on the Georgia coast', *Current Anthropology* 22, 137–148.

Larsen, C. S. (2012) 'Dietary reconstruction and nutritional assessment of past peoples: the bioanthropological record', in K. F. Kiple and C. O. Kriemhild (eds), *The Cambridge World History of Food*. Cambridge: Cambridge University Press, pp. 13–34.

Laureus (2010) *Teenage Kicks: The Value of Sport in Tackling Youth Crime*. London: Laureus Sport for Good Foundation.

Layard, R. (2005) *Happiness: Lessons from a New Science*. London: Penguin.

Leake, J. (2014) 'Polluted city air stunts babies' lungs in womb', *Sunday Times* (29 June), p. 2.

Lee, I-M., Shiroma, E., Lobelo, F., Puska, P., Blair, S. and Katzmarzyk, P. (2012) 'Effect of physical inactivity on major non-communicable diseases worldwide: an analysis of burden of disease and life expectancy', *The Lancet* 380(9838), 219–229. DOI: 10.1016/S0140-6736(12)61031-9

Lee, R. and Daly, R. (eds) (1999) *Cambridge History of Hunter Gatherers*. Cambridge: Cambridge University Press.

Lefebvre, H. (1991) *The Production of Space*, tr. D. Nicholson-Smith. Oxford: Blackwell.

Levin, N., Haile-Selassie, Y., Frost, S. and Saylor, B. (2015) 'Dietary change among hominins and cercopithecids in Ethiopia during the early Pliocene', *Proceedings of the National Academy of Sciences of the United States of America* 112(40), 12304–12309. DOI: 10.1073/pnas.1424982112

Lewis, M. C., Inman, C. F., Patel, D. V., Schmidt, B., Mulder, I., Miller, B. G. et al. (2012) 'Direct experimental evidence that early-life farm environment influences regulation of immune responses', *Pediatric Allergy and Immunology* 23(3), 265–269.

Lewis, R. A. (1952) *Edwin Chadwick and the Public Health Movement 1832–1854*. London: Longmans, Green.

Liebenberg, L. (2008) 'The relevance of persistence hunting to human evolution', *Journal of Human Evolution* 55(6), 1156–1159.

Lieberman, D., Werbel, W. and Daoud, A. (2009) 'Biomechanics of foot strike in habitually barefoot versus shod runners', *American Journal of Physical Anthropology* 208, 175–176.

Lim, S., Vos, T., Flaxman, A., Danaei, G., Shibuya, K., Adair-Rohani, H. et al. (2012) 'A comparative risk assessment of burden of disease and injury attributable to 67 risk factors and risk factor clusters in 21 regions, 1990–2010: a systematic analysis for the Global Burden of Disease Study 2010', *The Lancet* 380(9859), 2224–2260.

Lindeberg, S. (2010) *Food and Western Disease: Health and Nutrition from an Evolutionary Perspective*. Ames, IA: Wiley-Blackwell.

Lindeberg, S. and Lundh, B. (1993) 'Apparent absence of stroke and ischaemic heart disease in a traditional Melanesian population: a clinical study in Kitava', *Journal of International Medicine* 233, 269–275.

Linden, S. and Grut, J. (2002) *The Healing Fields: Working with Psychotherapy and Nature to Rebuild Shattered Lives*. London: Frances Lincoln.

Ling, L., Schneider, T., Peoples, A., Spoering, A., Engels, I., Conlon, B. et al. (2015) 'A new antibiotic kills pathogens without detectable resistance', *Nature* 517(7535), 455–459. DOI: 10.1038/nature14098

London Assembly Environment Committee (2006) *A Lot to Lose: London's Disappearing Allotments*. London: London Assembly Environment Committee.

Lustig, R. (2013) *Fat Chance: Beating the Odds Against Sugar, Processed Food, Obesity and Disease*. New York: Hudson.

Lyell, C. (1830–1833) *Principles of Geology, Being An Attempt to Explain the Former Changes of the Earth's Surface, By Reference to Causes Now in Operation*, 3 vols. London: John Murray.

Maas, J., Verheij, R., de Vries, S., Spreeuwenberg, P., Schellevis, F. and Groenewegen, P. (2009) 'Morbidity is related to a green living environment', *Journal of Epidemiology and Community Health* 63(12), 967–973. DOI: 10.1136/jech.2008.079038

Macfadyen, N. (2013) *Health and Garden Cities*. Town and Country Planning Tomorrow Series Paper 14. London: Town and Country Planning Association. (Re-publication of the Garden Cities and Town Planning Association pamphlet on the health benefits of garden cities, orig. pub. 1938.)

Magilton, J. (1980) *The Church of St Helen-on-the-Walls, Aldwark*. Archaeology of York 10/1. York: Council for British Archaeology.

Mahmood, S., Levy, D., Vasan, R. and Wang, T. (2014) 'The Framingham Heart Study and the epidemiology of cardiovascular disease: a historical perspective', *The Lancet* 383(9921), 999–1008. Available at: http://dx.doi.org/10.1016/S0140-6736(13)61752-3.

Malhotra, A., Apps, A. and Capewell, S. (2015) 'Maximising the benefits and minimising the harms of statins', *Prescriber* 26(1–2), 6–7. DOI: 10.1002/psb.1293

Marmot, M. G. (2010) *Fair Society, Healthy Lives: A Strategic Review of Health Inequalities in England Post-2010* (The Marmot Review). Available at: http://www.instituteofhealthequity. org/resources-reports/fair-society-healthy-lives-the-marmot-review.

Marmot, M. G. and Wilkinson, R. G. (eds) (2006) *Social Determinants of Health*. Oxford: Oxford University Press.

Marshall, S., Milne, G., Rook, G. and Tinnerman, R. (2015) 'Walking: a step-change towards healthy cities', *Town and Country Planning Journal* (March), 125–129.

Martin, A., Goryakin, Y. and Suhrcke, M. (2014) 'Does active commuting improve psychological wellbeing? Longitudinal evidence from eighteen waves of the British Household Panel Survey', *Preventive Medicine* 69, 296–303.

Michie, S., West, R., Campbell, R., Brown, J. and Gainforth, H. (2014) *ABC of Behaviour Change Theory: An Essential Reference for Researchers, Policy Makers and Practitioners*. Sutton: Silverback Publishing.

Milne, G. (1986) *The Great Fire of London*. London: Historical Publications.

Milne, G. (1990) 'King Alfred's plan for London?' *London Archaeologist* 6(8), 206–207.

Milne, G. (1996) 'Why is there nothing like a real fire?' *British Archaeology* 13 (April).

Milne, G. (1997) *St Bride's Church London: Archaeological Research 1952–60 and 1992–5*. English Heritage Archaeological Report 11. London: English Heritage.

Milne, G. (2002) *Excavations at Medieval Cripplegate, London: Archaeology After the Blitz*. London: English Heritage.

Milne, G. (2015) 'The Evolutionary Determinants of Health Programme: urban living in the 21st century from a human evolutionary perspective', *Archaeology International* 18, 84–96.

Milton, K. (1999a) 'A hypothesis to explain the role of meat-eating in human evolution', *Evolutionary Anthropology* 8, 11–21.

Milton, K. (1999b) 'Nutritional characteristics of wild primate foods: do the natural diets of our closest living relatives have lessons for us?' *Nutrition* 15(6), 488–498.

Milton, K. (1999c) 'Commentary on cooking and the ecology of human origins', *Current Anthropology* 40, 583–584.

Milton, K. (2000a) 'Back to basics: why foods of wild primates have relevance for modern human health', *Nutrition* 16, 481–483.

Milton, K. (2000b) 'Hunter-gatherer diets: a different perspective', *American Journal of Clinical Nutrition* 71, 665–667.

Minger, D. (2013) *Death by Food Pyramid*. Malibu, CA: Primal Blueprint Publishing.

Mirazón Lahr, M., Rivera, F., Power, R., Mounier, A., Copsey, B., Crivellaro, F. et al. (2016) 'Inter-group violence among early Holocene hunter-gatherers of West Turkana, Kenya', *Nature* 529, 394–398. DOI: 10.1038/nature16477

Mitchell, R. and Popham, F. (2008) 'Effect of exposure to natural environment on health inequalities: an observational population study', *The Lancet* 372(9650), 1655–1660.

Mithen, S. J. (1996) *The Prehistory of the Mind: A Search for the Origins of Art, Religion, and Science*. London: Thames & Hudson.

Mithen, S. J. (2005) *The Singing Neanderthals: The Origins of Music, Language, Mind and Body*. London: Weidenfeld and Nicolson.

Monbiot, G. (2013) *Feral: Searching for Enchantment on the Frontiers of Rewilding*. London: Penguin.

Monboddo, J. B., Lord (1774) *Of the Origin and Progress of Language*. Edinburgh: Printed for J. Balfour.

Morgan, L. (1877) *Ancient Society; Or, Researches in the Lines of Human Progress from Savagery through Barbarism to Civilisation*. New York: H. Holt and Co.

Morgan, M. H. (1960 [1914]) *Vitruvius: The Ten Books on Architecture*. New York: Dover.

Morris, D. (1967) *The Naked Ape: A Zoologist's Study of the Human Animal*. London: Jonathan Cape.

Morris, D. (1969) *The Human Zoo*. London: Jonathan Cape.

Morris, J., Heady, J., Raffle, P., Roberts, C. and Parks, J. (1953a) 'Coronary heart-disease and physical activity of work', *The Lancet* 2, 1053–1057.

Morris, J., Heady, J., Raffle, P., Roberts, C. and Parks, J. (1953b) 'Coronary heart-disease and physical activity of work', *The Lancet* 2, 1111–1120.

Morris, R. (1989) *Churches in the Landscape*. London: J.M. Dent & Sons.

Morris, T. (2007) 'Social and therapeutic horticulture at a boys' special residential school', *Growth Point – The Journal of Social and Therapeutic Horticulture* 110, 9–11.

Mostafavi, M. and Doherty, G. (2010) *Ecological Urbanism*. Baden: Lars Muller.

Mostafavi, M. and Najle, C. (eds) (2004) *Landscape Urbanism: A Manual for the Machinic Landscape*. London: Architectural Association.

Mujcic, R. (2014) 'Are fruit and vegetables good for our mental and physical health? Panel data evidence from Australia'. Munich Personal RePEc Archive paper no. 59149. Available at: http://mpra.ub.uni-muenchen.de/59149/1/MPRA_paper_59149.pdf.

Nature (2005) 'The chimpanzee genome', *Nature* 437, 48–49. Available at: http://www.nature.com/nature/journal/v437/n7055/full/437048a.html.

Neel, J. (1962) 'Diabetes mellitus: a "thrifty" genotype rendered detrimental by "progress"?' *American Journal of Human Genetics* 14(4), 353.

NHS (n.d.) 'Eight tips for healthy eating', *NHS*. Available at: http://www.nhs.uk/Livewell/Goodfood/Pages/eight-tips-healthy-eating.aspx.

NICE (2006) *Public Health Guidance: Obesity Prevention NICE Guidelines CG43* [now under review]. London: National Institute for Health and Care Excellence.

NICE (2007) *Public Health Guideline 6: Behaviour Change: General Approaches*. London: National Institute for Health and Care Excellence.

NICE (2008a) *Public Health Guidance 8: Physical Activity and the Environment*. London: National Institute for Health and Care Excellence.

NICE (2008b) *Public Health Guidance 13: Promoting Physical Activity in the Work Place*. London: National Institute for Health and Care Excellence.

NICE (2009) *Public Health Guidance 17: Promoting Physical Activity for Children and Young People*. London: National Institute for Health and Care Excellence.

NICE (2010) *Public Health Guidance 25: Prevention of Cardiovascular Disease*. London: National Institute for Health and Care Excellence.

NICE (2012) *Public Health Guidance 41: Walking and Cycling: Local Measures to Promote Walking and Cycling as Forms of Travel or Recreation*. London: National Institute for Health and Care Excellence.

NICE (2015) *National Guidelines 7: Preventing Excess Weight Gain*. London: National Institute for Health and Care Excellence.

NICE (2016) *NICE Guidelines 34: Sunlight Exposure: Risks and Benefits*. London: National Institute for Health and Care Excellence.

NIDDK (2014) 'Lactose intolerance', *National Institute of Diabetes and Digestive and Kidney Diseases*. Available at: https://www.niddk.nih.gov/health-information/health-topics/digestive-diseases/lactose-intolerance/Pages/facts.aspx.

O'Keefe, J. and Cordain, L. (2004) 'Cardiovascular disease resulting from a diet and lifestyle at odds with our Palaeolithic genome: how to become a 21st-century hunter-gatherer', *Mayo Clinic Proceedings* 79, 101–108.

O'Keefe, J., Vogel, R., Lavie, C. and Cordain, L. (2011) 'Exercise like a hunter-gatherer: a prescription for organic physical fitness', *Progress in Cardiovascular Diseases* 53, 471–479.

Oakes, B. (1995) *Sculpting with the Environment*. New York: Van Nostrand Reinhold.

OECD (2013) *How's Life? 2013. Measuring Well-Being. Country Snapshot: France*. Paris: Organisation for Economic Co-operation and Development. Available at: http://www.oecd.org/fr/statistiques/HsL-Country-Note-France-Fr.pdf.

ONS (2012) *Measuring National Well-Being: First Annual Report on Measuring National Well-Being, 2012*. Newport: Office for National Statistics.

ONS (2013a) *Healthy Life Expectancy at Birth for Upper Tier Local Authorities, England: 2010 to 2012*. Newport: Office for National Statistics. Available at: https://www.ons.gov.uk/peoplepopulationandcommunity/healthandsocialcare/healthandlifeexpectancies/bulletins/healthylifeexpectancyatbirthforuppertierlocalauthoritiesengland/2014-07-18#summary.

ONS (2013b) *Local Authority Variations in Self-Assessed General Health for Males and Females, England and Wales, 2011*. Newport: Office for National Statistics.

Ornish, D. (1993) *Eat More, Weigh Less*. New York: HarperCollins.

Oyebode, O., Gordon-Dseagu, V., Walker, A. and Mindell, J. (2014) 'Fruit and vegetable consumption and all-cause, cancer and CVD mortality: analysis of Health Survey for England data', *Journal of Epidemiology and Community Health* 68(9), 856–862. DOI: 10.1136/jech-2013-203500

Ozer, E. J. (2007) 'The effects of school gardens on students and schools: conceptualisation and considerations for maximizing healthy development', *Health Education and Behaviour* 34(6), 846–863.

Pääbo, S. (2014) *Neanderthal Man: In Search of Lost Genomes*. New York: Basic Books.

Parr, H. (2005) Sustainable Communities? Nature Work and Mental Health. University of Dundee, Economic and Social Research Council.

Patten, M. (1985) *We'll Eat Again: A Collection of Recipes from the War Years*. London: Hamlyn.

Patterson, N., Richter, D., Gnerre, S., Lander, E. and Reich, D. (2006) 'Genetic evidence for complex speciation of humans and chimpanzees', *Nature* 441, 1103–1108. DOI: 10.1038/nature04789

Pearse, I. and Crocker, L. (1943) *The Peckham Experiment: A Study of the Living Structure of Society*. London: George Allen and Unwin.

Peter, H. and Kahn, J. R. (1997) 'Developmental psychology and the biophilia hypothesis: children's affiliation with nature', *Developmental Review* 17, 1–61.

Pevsner, N. (1973) *The Buildings of England*. Vol. 1: *The City of London*. New Haven, CT and London: Yale University Press.

PHE and LGA (2013) *Obesity and the Environment: Increasing Physical Activity and Active Travel*. London: Public Health England and the Local Government Association.

Pinker, S. (1997) *How the Mind Works*. New York: Norton.

Pinto Pereira, S., Geoffroy, M. and Power, C. (2014) 'Depressive symptoms and physical activity during 3 decades in adult life: bidirectional associations in a prospective cohort study', *JAMA Psychiatry* 71(12), 1373–1380. DOI: 10.1001/jamapsychiatry.2014.1240

Pitts, M. and Roberts, M. (1998) *Fairweather Eden: Life in Britain Half a Million Years Ago as Revealed by the Excavations at Boxgrove*. London: Arrow.

Pluciennik, M. (2005) *Social Evolution*. London: Duckworth.

Poole, C. G. (2012) Making Walking and Cycling Normal: Key Findings from the Understanding Walking and Cycling Research Project. Unpublished report for NICE, Lancaster Environment Centre, Lancaster University.

Popkin, B., Adair, L. and Ng, S. (2012) 'Global nutrition transition and the pandemic of obesity in developing countries', *Nutrition Reviews* 70, 3–21.

Pretty, J., Griffin, M., Peacock, J., Hine, R., Sellens, M. and South, N. (2005) *A Countryside for Health and Wellbeing: The Physical and Mental Health Benefits of Green Exercise*. Sheffield: Countryside Recreation Network.

Price, W. (1939) *Nutrition and Physical Degeneration: A Comparison of the Primitive and Modern Diet and Their Effects*. Redlands, CA: Published by author.

Punter, J. (2011) 'Urban design and the English urban renaissance 1999–2009: a review and preliminary evaluation', *Journal of Urban Design* 16(1), 1–41.

Quayle, H. (2008) *The True Value of Community Farms and Gardens: Social, Environmental, Health and Economic*. Bristol: Federation of City Farms and Community Gardens.

Rahm, J. (2002) 'Emergent learning opportunities in an inner-city youth gardening program', *Journal of Research Science in Teaching* 39(2), 164–184.

Ratey, J. and Manning, R. (2014) *Go Wild: Free Your Body and Mind from the Afflictions of Civilisation*. New York: Little, Brown and Co.

Reddaway, T. F. (1940) *The Rebuilding of London after the Great Fire*. London: Jonathan Cape.

Reich, D., Green, R. and Pääbo, S. (2010) 'Genetic history of an archaic hominin group from Denisova Cave in Siberia', *Nature* 468, 1053–1060.

Reinhard, K. J. (2000) 'Coprolite analysis: the analysis of ancient human feces for dietary data', in L. Ellis (ed.), *Archaeological Method and Theory: An Encyclopedia*. New York and London: Garland Publishing, pp. 124–132.

Reinhard, K. J. and Bryant, V. M. (2008) 'Pathoecology and the future of coprolite studies', in A. W. M. Stodder (ed.), *Reanalysis and Reinterpretation in Southwestern Bioarchaeology*. Tempe, AZ: Arizona State University Press, pp. 199–216.

Reinhard, K. J., Ferreira, L., Bouchet, F., Sianto, L., Dutra, L., Iniguez, A., Leles, D., Le Bailly, M., Fugassa, M., Pucu, E. and Araújo, A. (2013) 'Food, parasites, and epidemiological transitions: a broad perspective', *International Journal of Paleopathology* 3(3), 150–157. Available at: http://digitalcommons.unl.edu/natresreinhard/15.

Reul, G., Shi, Z., Zhen, S., Zuo, H., Kröger, E., Sirois, C., Lévesque, J. F. and Taylor, A. W. (2013) 'The association between nutrition and the evolution of multimorbidity: the importance of fruits and vegetables and whole grain products', *Clinical Nutrition* 33(5), 513–520.

Richards, S. (2005) 'Maintaining independence in old age: the importance of domestic gardens and gardening', *Growth Point – Journal of Social and Therapeutic Horticulture* 101, 10–11.

Ridsdale, B. and Gallop, A. (2010) 'Mortality by cause of death and by socio-economic and demographic stratification 2010'. Paper for International Actuarial Association. Ref: 183_paper_Ridsdale, Gallop.

Rightmire, P. (2009) 'Out of Africa: modern human origins special feature: middle and later Pleistocene hominins in Africa and Southwest Asia', *Proceedings of the National Academy of Sciences of the USA* 106, 16046–16050.

Roberts, C. and Cox, M. (2003) *Health and Disease in Britain, from Prehistory to the Present Day*. Stroud: Sutton Publishing.

Roberts, L., Ashmore, T., Kotwica, A., Murfitt, S., Fernandez, B., Feelisch, M., Murray, A. and Griffin, J. (2015) 'Inorganic nitrate promotes the browning of white adipose tissue through the nitrate-nitrite-nitric oxide pathway', *Diabetes* 64(2), 471–484. DOI: 10.2337/db14-0496

Roberts, M. B. and Parfitt, S. A. (1999) *Boxgrove: A Middle Pleistocene Hominid Site at Eartham Quarry, Boxgrove, West Sussex*. London: English Heritage.

Robertson, A., Brunner, E. and Sheiham, A. (2005) 'Food is a political issue', in M. G. Marmot and R. G. Wilkinson (eds), *Social Determinants of Health*. Oxford: Oxford University Press, pp. 179–201.

Robertson, G. (2007) 'Gardening at the Thomas Tallis School learning support unit', *Growth Point – Journal of Social and Therapeutic Horticulture* 110, 13–16.

Rodwell, W. and Rodwell, K. (1982) 'St Peter's Church, Barton on Humber', *Antiquaries Journal* 62, 283–315.

Rong, Y., Chen, L., Zhu, T., Song, Y., Yu, M., Shan, Z., Sands, A., Hu, F. B. and Liu, L. (2013) 'Egg consumption and risk of coronary heart disease and stroke: dose-response meta-analysis of prospective cohort studies', *BMJ* 346: e8539. DOI: 10.1136/bmj.e8539

Rook, G. (2012) 'Hygiene hypothesis and autoimmune diseases', *Clinical Reviews in Allergy & Immunology* 42(4), 1–15.

Rook, G. (2013) 'Regulation of the immune system by biodiversity from the natural environment: an ecosystem service essential to health', *Proceedings of the National Academy of Sciences of the United States of America* 110(46), 18360–18367. DOI: 10.1073/pnas.1313731110

Rook, G., Raison, C. and Lowry, C. (2013) 'Childhood microbial experience, immunoregulation, inflammation and adult susceptibility to psychosocial stressors and depression in rich and poor countries', *Evolution, Medicine, and Public Health* 1, 14–17. DOI: 10.1093/emph/eos005

Rook, G., Raison, C. and Lowry, C. (2014) 'Microbial "old friends", immunoregulation and socio-economic status', *Clinical and Experimental Immunology* 177, 13–23. DOI: 101111/cei.12269

Rosengren, A., Anderson, K. and Wilhelmsen, L. (1991) 'Risk of coronary heart disease in middle-aged male bus and tram drivers', *International Journal of Epidemiology* 20, 82–87.

RSI Therapy (2005) 'RSI statistics'. Available at: http://www.rsi-therapy.com/statistics.htm.

Ruano, M. (1998) *Eco-Urbanism: Sustainable Human Settlements, 60 Case Studies*. Barcelona: Gustavo Gili.

Rubino, F., Nathan, D. M., Eckel, R. H., Schauer, P. R., Alberti, K. G., Zimmet, P. Z. et al. (2016) 'Metabolic surgery in the treatment algorithm for type 2 diabetes: a joint statement by international diabetes organizations', *Diabetes Care* 39, 861–877.

Ruel, G., Zumin, S., Zhem, S., Zuo, H., Kröger, E., Sirois, C., Lévesque, J. and Taylor, A. (2013) 'Association between nutrition and the evolution of multimorbidity: the importance of fruits and vegetables and whole grain products', *Journal of Clinical Nutrition* 33(3), 513–520.

Ruff, C., Holt, B., Niskanenc, M., Sladekd, V., Bernere, M., Garofalof, E., Garving, H., Horad, M., Junnoc, J., Schuplerovad, E., Vilkamac, R. and Whittey, E. (2015) 'Gradual decline in mobility with the adoption of food production in Europe', *Proceedings of the National Academy of Sciences of the United States of America* 112(23), 7147–7152. DOI: 10.1073/pnas.1502932112

Ryan, T. and Shaw, C. (2014) 'Gracility of the modern Homo sapiens skeleton is the result of decreased biomechanical loading', *Proceedings of the National Academy of Sciences of the United States of America* 112(2), 372–377. DOI: 10.1073/pnas1418646112

Rydin, Y., Bleahu, A., Davies, M., Groce, N., Scott, I. and Wilkinson, P. (2012) 'Shaping cities for health: complexity and the planning of urban environments in the 21st century', *The Lancet* 379(9831), 2079–2108.

SACN (2015) *Carbohydrates and Health. Scientific Advisory Committee on Nutrition 2015.* London: TSO.

Samuels, J., Bienvenu, O., Grados, M., Cullen, B., Riddle, M., Liang, K., Eaton, W. and Nestadt, G. (2008) 'Prevalence and correlates of hoarding behavior in a community-based sample', *Behaviour Research and Therapy* 46: 836–844.

Schrire, C. (ed.) (1984) *Past and Present in Hunter-Gatherer Studies.* New York: Academic Press.

Schumacher, E. F. (1973) *Small is Beautiful: A Study of Economics As If People Mattered.* London: Blond & Briggs.

Sempik, J. and Aldridge, J. (2006) 'Care farms and care gardens: horticulture as therapy in the UK', in J. Hassink and M. van Dijk (eds), *Farming for Health: Green-Care Farming Across Europe and the United States of America.* Dordrecht: Springer, pp. 147–161.

Sempik, J., Aldridge, J. and Becker, S. (2003a) *Social and Therapeutic Horticulture: Evidence and Messages from Research.* Evidence Issue 6. Loughborough: Thrive and the Centre for Child and Family Research, Loughborough University.

Sempik, J., Aldridge, J. and Becker, S. (2003b) 'Treating the maniacs? Horticulture as a therapy: from Benjamin Rush to the present day'. Draft paper presented at Horticultural Geographies Conference, Nottingham University.

Sempik, J., Aldridge, J. and Finnis, L. (2004) *Social and Therapeutic Horticulture: The State of Practice in the UK.* Evidence Issue 8. Loughborough: Centre for Child and Family Research, Loughborough University.

Seymour, J. (1976) *The Complete Book of Self-Sufficiency.* London: Faber & Faber.

Shane, D. (2003) 'The emergence of "landscape urbanism"', *Harvard Design Magazine* 19 (Fall/Winter).

Shennan, S. (2003) *Genes, Memes and Human History: Darwinian Archaeology and Cultural Evolution.* London: Thames & Hudson.

Shennan, S. (2011) 'An evolutionary perspective on the goals of archaeology', in E. Cochrane and A. Gardner (eds), *Evolutionary and Interpretive Archaeologies: A Dialogue.* Walnut Creek, CA: Left Coast Press, pp. 325–344.

Shennan, S., Downey, S., Timpson, A., Edinborough, K., Colledge, S., Kerig, T., Manning, K. and Thomas, M. G. (2013) 'Regional population collapse followed initial agriculture booms in mid-Holocene Europe', *Nature Communications.* Available at: http://www.nature.com/articles/ncomms3486.

Shorta, M. B., Brantingham, P. J., Bertozzic, A. L. and Titad, G. E. (2010) 'Dissipation and displacement of hotspots in reaction-diffusion models of crime', *Proceedings of the National Academy of Sciences of the United States of America* 107(9), 3961–3965. Available at: http://www.pnas.org/content/107/9/3961.full.

Sibley, C. and Ahlquist, J. (1984) 'The phylogeny of the hominoid primates, as indicated by DNA-DNA hybridization', *Journal of Molecular Evolution* 20(1), 2–15.

Simopoulos, A. (ed.) (1999) *Evolutionary Aspects of Nutrition and Health: Diet, Exercise, Genetics and Chronic Disease*, Vol. 84. Basel: Karger.

Simopoulos, A. (2000) 'Human requirement for n-3 polyunsaturated fatty acids', *Poultry Science* 79(7), 961–970.

Simopoulos, A. (2006) 'Evolutionary aspects of diet, the omega-6/omega-3 ration and genetic variation: nutritional implications for chronic diseases', *Biomedicine and Pharmacotherapy* 60, 502–507.

Simopoulos, A. and Robinson, J. (1998) *The Omega Diet.* New York: HarperCollins.

Sissons, M. (2009) *The Primal Blueprint: Reprogramme Your Genes for Effortless Weight Loss, Vibrant Health and Boundless Energy.* Malibu, CA: Primal Nutrition.

Sobolik, K. D. (2012) 'Dietary reconstruction as seen in coprolites', in K. F. Kiple and C. O. Kriemhild (eds), *The Cambridge World History of Food*. Cambridge: Cambridge University Press, pp. 44–51.

Song, M. and Giovannucci, E. (2016) 'Preventable incidence and mortality of carcinoma associated with lifestyle factors among white adults in the United States', *JAMA Oncology* 2(9), 1154–1161. DOI: 10.1001/jamaoncol.2016.0843

Stamatakis, E., Chau, J., Pedisic, Z., Bauman, A., Macniven, R., Coombs, N. and Mamer, M. (2013) 'Are sitting occupations associated with increased all-cause mortality, cancer and cardiovascular disease mortality risk?' *PLOS ONE* 8(9): e73753.

Stanford, C. (1999) *The Hunting Apes: Meat Eating and the Origins of Human Behavior*. Princeton, NJ: Princeton University Press.

Stanford, C. and Bunn, H. (eds) (2001) *Meat-Eating and Human Evolution* (Human Evolution Series). Oxford: Oxford University Press.

Stefansson, V. (1946) *Not by Bread Alone*. New York: Macmillan.

Stiglitz, J., Sen, A. and Fitoussi, J. (2010) *Mismeasuring Our Lives: Why GDP Doesn't Add Up: The Report*. New York: New Press.

Stiner, M., Gopher, A. and Barkai, R. (2010) 'Hearth-side socioeconomics, hunting and paleoecology during the late Lower Paleolithic at Qesem Cave, Israel', *Journal of Human Evolution* 30, 1–21.

Stringer, C. (2006) *Homo Britannicus: The Incredible Story of Human Life in Britain*. London: Penguin.

Stringer, C. and Andrews, P. (2011) *The Complete Word of Human Evolution*. London: Thames & Hudson.

Sundquist, K., Frank, G. and Sundquist, J. (2004) 'Urbanisation and incidence of psychosis and depression: follow-up study of 4.4 million women and men in Sweden', *British Journal of Psychiatry* 184, 293–298.

Sustrans (2009) 'Why walk? Step your way to a happy, healthy lifestyle'. Available at: http://www.north-ayrshire.gov.uk/Documents/CorporateServices/LegalProtective/LocalDevelopmentPlan/WhyWalk.pdf.

Tamosiunas, A., Grazuleviciene, R., Luksiene, D., Dedele, A., Reklaitiene, R., Baceviciene, M., Vencloviene, J., Bernotiene, G., Radisauskas, R., Malinauskiene, V., Milinaviciene, E., Bobak, M., Peasey, A. and Nieuwenhuijsen, J. (2014) 'Accessibility and use of urban green spaces and cardiovascular health: findings from a Kaunas cohort study', *Environmental Health* 13(1), 20. DOI: 10.1186/1476-069X-13-20

Taylor, A. F., Kuo, F. and Sullivan, W. C. (2001) 'Coping with ADD: the surprising connection to green play settings', *Environment and Behaviour* 33, 54–77.

Tedstone, A. (2016) 'Sugar reduction and obesity: 10 things you need to know', *Public Health England* (1 November). Available at: https://publichealthmatters.blog.gov.uk/2016/11/01/sugar-reduction-and-obesity-10-things-you-need-to-know/.

TfL (2014) *Improving the Health of Londoners: Transport Action Plan*. London: Transport for London.

Thayer, R. (1994) *Gray World, Green Heart: Technology, Nature and the Sustainable Landscape*. New York: John Wiley and Sons.

Thomas, H. (2012) 'Ten tenets and six questions for landscape urbanism', *Landscape Research* 37(1), 7–26.

Thomsen, C. J. (1848) *Guide to Northern Antiquities*. London: James Bain.

Tooby, J. and Cosmides, L. (2005) 'Conceptual foundations of evolutionary psychology', in D. M. Buss (ed.), *The Handbook of Evolutionary Psychology*. Hoboken, NJ: Wiley, pp. 5–67.

Treib, M. (1993) *Modern Landscape Architecture: A Critical Review*. Cambridge, MA: MIT Press.

Trowell, H. and Burkitt, D. (1981) *Western Diseases: The Emergence and Prevention*. Cambridge, MA: Harvard University Press.

Tse, J. L., Flin, R. and Mearns, K. (2006) 'Bus driver well-being review: 50 years of research', *Transportation Research Part F* 9, 89–114.

Tsouros, A. (1990) *Healthy Cities Project: A Project Becomes a Movement*. Copenhagen: FADL Publishers for the WHO Healthy Cities Project Office.

Turner, T. (2010) 'What is landscape urbanism?' *Garden Visit* (February). Available at: http://www.gardenvisit.com/blog/2010/02/.

Tykot, R. (2004) 'Stable isotopes and diet: you are what you eat', in M. Martini, M. Milazzo and M. Piacentini (eds), *Physics Methods in Archaeometry. Vol. 154 of the Proceedings of the International School of Physics 'Enrico Fermi' Course CLIV*. Amsterdam: IOS Press, pp. 433–444.

UCL (2015) 'International UCL-led study prompts rethink on the rise of diabetes in cities', *University College London* (16 November). Available at: http://www.ucl.ac.uk/consultants/uclc-news/diabetes.

Ulrich, R. (1984) 'View through a window may influence recovery from surgery', *American Association for the Advancement of Science, New Series* 224(4647), 420–421.

UN-DESA (2012) *World Urbanization Prospects: The 2011 Revision*. New York: United Nations Department of Economics and Social Affairs. Available at: http://www.un.org/en/development/desa/population/publications/pdf/urbanization/WUP2011_Report.pdf.

UN-DESA (2015) *The World Population Prospects: 2015 Revision*. New York: United Nations Department of Economics and Social Affairs. Available at: https://esa.un.org/unpd/wpp/Publications/Files/Key_Findings_WPP_2015.pdf.

UN-HABITAT (2008) *State of the World's Cities 2008/2009: Harmonious Cities*. London and Washington, DC: Earthscan.

UNDP (1990) *Human Development Report 1990*. New York and Oxford: Oxford University Press (for the United Nations Development Programme).

Ungar, P. S. (ed.) (2006) *Evolution of the Human Diet*. Oxford: Oxford University Press.

University of Exeter (2013) 'Office plants boost well-being at work' (press release, 9 July). Available at: http://www.exeter.ac.uk/news/research/title_306119_en.html.

Unwin, G. (1908) *The Gilds and Companies of London*. London: Methuen & Co.

USDA (2015) *Scientific Report of the 2015 Dietary Guidelines Advisory Committee: Advisory Report to the Secretary of Health and Human Services and the Secretary of Agriculture*. Washington, DC: United States Department of Agriculture.

Vanna, V. (2007) 'Sex and gender related health status differences in ancient and contemporary skeletal populations', *Papers from the UCL Institute of Archaeology* 18, 114–147.

Velde, B. P., Cipriani, J. and Fisher, G. (2005) 'Resident and therapist views of animal assisted therapy: implications for occupational therapy practice', *Australian Occupational Therapy Journal* 52, 43–50.

Voegtlin, W. (1975) *The Stone Age Diet*. New York: Vantage Press.

von Mutius, E. and Vercelli, D. (2010) 'Farm living: effects on childhood asthma and allergy', *Nature Reviews Immunology* 10(12), 861–868. DOI: 10.1038/nri2871

Waldheim, C. (ed.) (2006) *The Landscape Urbanism Reader*. New York: Princeton Architectural Press.

Waldheim, C. (2010) 'On landscape, ecology and other modifiers to urbanism', *Topos* 71, 20–24.

Wale, M. (2004) 'The history of London allotments: the need for growing food in London and the role of the allotment in London's future'. Speech to the Greater London Allotments Forum (GLAF), City Hall, London, 23 July.

Wallin, N., Merker, B. and Brown, S. (2000) *The Origins of Music*. Cambridge, MA: MIT Press.

Wang, P. and Lin, R. (2001) 'Coronary heart disease risk factors in urban bus drivers', *Public Health* 115, 261–264.

Wanless, D. (2002) 'Securing our future health: taking a long-term view' – Final report, London: HM Treasury. Available at: http://www.yearofcare.co.uk/sites/default/files/images/Wanless.pdf.

Watts, M. (2016) 'Emeli Sande: I'll go into jails to sing with young offenders', *Evening Standard* (4 March), p. 13.

Webb, O. and Eves, J. (2006) 'Promoting stair climbing: effects of message', *Health Education Research* 22, 49–57. DOI: 10.1093/her/cyl045

Webb, O. and Eves, F. (2007) 'Promoting stair-climbing: intervention effects generalize to a subsequent stair ascent', *American Journal of Health Promotion* 22, 114–119. Available at: http://dx.doi.org/10.4278/0890-1171-22.2.114.

Weiner, A. (1988) *The Trobrianders of Papua New Guinea* (Case Studies in Cultural Anthropology). Sunrise, FL: Holt, Rinehart and Winston.

Wells, J. (2016) *The Metabolic Ghetto: An Evolutionary Perspective on Nutrition, Power Relations and Chronic Disease*. Cambridge: Cambridge University Press.

Welsh Government (2016) *An Active Travel Action Plan for Wales*. Available at: http://gov.wales/docs/det/publications/160229-active-travel-action-plan-wales-en.pdf.

WGBC (2013) *Business Case for Green Building*. World Green Building Council.

Wheatley, H. B. (ed.) (1956) *Stow's Survey of London*. London: J.M. Dent & Sons.

White, M. P., Alcock, I., Wheeler, B. W. and Depledge, M. H. (2013a) 'Coastal proximity, health and well-being: results from a longitudinal panel survey', *Health and Place* 23, 97–103.

White, M. P., Alcock, I., Wheeler, B. W. and Depledge, M. H. (2013b) 'Would you be happier living in a greener urban area? A fixed-effects analysis of panel data', *Psychological Science* 24(6), 920–928.

White, T. D., Asfaw, B., Beyene, Y., Haile-Selassie, Y., Lovejoy, C., Suwa, G. and Wolde, G. (2009) '*Ardipithecus ramidus* and the paleobiology of early hominids', *Science* 326(5949), 75–86.

Whitelock, D. (ed.) (1979) *English Historical Documents. Vol. 1: c.500–1040*. London: Eyre & Spottiswoode.

WHO (1990) *Diet, Nutrition, and the Prevention of Chronic Diseases* (Technical Report Series 797). Geneva: World Health Organization.

WHO (2004) *The Global Burden of Disease: 2004 Update*. Geneva: World Health Organization.

WHO (2015) *Guideline: Sugars Intake for Adults and Children*. Geneva: World Health Organization.

WHO (2016) *Global Report on Diabetes*. Geneva: World Health Organization. Available at: http://apps.who.int/iris/bitstream/10665/204871/1/9789241565257_eng.pdf.

WHO and UNICEF (2010) *Progress on Sanitation and Drinking-Water: An Update*. Geneva and New York: World Health Organization and UNICEF.

Wilby, R. L. and Perry, G. (2006) 'Climate change, biodiversity and the urban environment: a critical review based on London, UK', *Progress in Physical Geography* 30, 73–98.

Wilson, E. O. (1981) *Genes, Mind and Culture*. Cambridge, MA: Harvard University Press.

Wilson, E. O. (1984) *Biophilia*. Cambridge, MA: Harvard University Press.

Wilson, E. O. (1998) *Consilience: The Unity of Knowledge*. New York: Alfred A. Knopf.

Winegard, B. and Deaner, R. O. (2010) 'The evolutionary significance of Red Sox nation: sport fandom as a by-product of coalitional psychology', *Evolutionary Psychology* 8(3), 432–446.

Wing, E. (2012) 'Animals used for food in the past as seen by their remains excavated from archaeological sites', in K. F. Kiple and C. O. Kriemhild (eds), *The Cambridge World History of Food*. Cambridge: Cambridge University Press, pp. 51–58.

Wing, E. and Brown, A. (1979) *Palaeo-Nutrition: Method and Theory in Prehistoric Foodways*. New York: Academic Press.

Wise, C., Palwyn, M. and Braungart, M. (2013) 'Eco-engineering in a materials world', *Nature* 494, 172–175.

Witchel, H. (2011) *You Are What You Hear: How Music and Territory Make Us Who We Are*. New York: Algora Publishing.

Wolpert, S. (2010) 'Can math and science help solve crimes? UCLA scientists work with L.A. police to identify and analyze crime "hotspots"', *UCLA Newsroom* (20 February). Available at: http://newsroom.ucla.edu/releases/can-math-and-science-help-solve-153986.

Wrangham, R. (2009) *Catching Fire: How Cooking Made Us Human*. London: Profile Books.

Wray, A. (2000a) *Formulaic Language and the Lexicon*. Cambridge: Cambridge University Press.

Wray, A. (2000b) 'Holistic utterances and proto language: the link from primates to humans', in C. Knight, M. Studdert-Kennedy and J. Hurford (eds), *The Evolutionary Emergence of Language: Social Function and the Origins of Linguistic Form*. Cambridge: Cambridge University Press, pp. 285–302.

Wray, A. (ed.) (2002) *The Transition to Language*. Cambridge: Cambridge University Press.

Wright, R. D. (1994) *The Moral Animal: The New Science of Evolutionary Psychology*. New York: Vintage.

Ye, K. and Gu, Z. (2011) 'Recent advances in understanding the role of nutrition in human genome evolution', *Advances in Nutrition: An International Review Journal* 2, 486–496.

Yerushalmy, J. and Hilleboe, H. (1957) 'Fat in the diet and mortality from heart disease: a methodological note', *New York State Journal of Medicine* 57(14), 2343–2354.

Yokoyama, Y., Barnard, N., Levin, S. and Watanabe, M. (2014) 'Vegetarian diets and glycemic control in diabetes: a systematic review and meta-analysis', *Cardiovascular Diagnosis and Therapy* 4(5), 373–382.

Yuan, C., Gaskins, A., Blaine, A., Zhang, C., Gillman, M., Missmer, S., Field, A. and Chavarro, J. (2016) 'Association between cesarean birth and risk of obesity in offspring in childhood, adolescence, and early adulthood', *JAMA Pediatrics*. Published online 6 September. DOI: 10.1001/jamapediatrics.2016.2385

Yudkin, J. (1963) 'Nutrition and palatability with special reference to obesity, myocardial infarction, and other diseases of civilisation', *The Lancet* 1(7295), 1335–1338. DOI: 10.1016/s0140-6736(63)91920-2

Yudkin, J. (2012 [1972]) *Pure, White and Deadly*. London: Penguin.

Zalasiewicz, J., Williams, M., Steffen, W. and Crutzen, P. (2010) 'The new world of the Anthropocene', *Environmental Science & Technology* 44(7), 2228–2231. DOI: 10.1021/es903118j

Zweiniger-Bargielowska, I. (2000) *Austerity in Britain: Rationing, Controls and Consumption 1939–1955*. Oxford: Oxford University Press.

INDEX

PICTURE CREDITS

Page 12, © Erica Guilane-Nachez, Fotolia

Page 15, © Morphart, Fotolia

Figure 2.1: page 23, © ruskpp, Fotolia

Page 26, © nickolae, Fotolia

Page 30, from *Evidence as to Man's Place in Nature*, T. Huxley (1863)

Figure 2.2: page 31, © Charlotte Frearson

Page 32, © UCL Creative Media Services

Figure 2.3: page 35, © nicholasprimola, Fotolia

Figure 2.4: page 35, © Charlotte Frearson

Figure 2.5: page 38, © Erica Guilane-Nachez, Fotolia

Figure 3.1: page 44, © Morphart, Fotolia

Page 49, © ruskpp, Fotolia

Figure 4.1: page 59, © Charlotte Frearson

Figure 4.2: page 60, (1), © Erica Guilane-Nachez, Fotolia, (2), © unorobus, Fotolia

Figure 4.3: page 64, (1), © acrogame, Fotolia, (2) © Morphart, Fotolia

Figure 4.4: page 65, © Erica Guilane-Nachez, Fotolia

Figure 5.1: page 73, © Erica Guilane-Nachez, Fotolia

Page 81, © Erica Guilane-Nachez, Fotolia

Page 95, © Morphart, Fotolia

Figure 6.1: page 96, © Charlotte Frearson

Figure 6.2: page 97, © acrogame, Fotolia

Figure 7.1: page 106, © Charlotte Frearson

Figure 8.1: page 116, © Erica Guilane-Nachez, Fotolia

Figure 8.2: page 119, © Erica Guilane-Nachez, Fotolia

Page 122: (1), © Morphant, Fotolia, (2), © Erica Guilane-Nachez, Fotolia, (3), © acrogame, Fotolia

Page 124, © Keene and Harding

Figure 9.1: page 132, (1), © Vasiliy Voropaev, Fotolia, (2), © Alexey Pavuts, Fotolia

Figure 10.1: page 139, (1), © Erica Guilane-Nachez, Fotolia, (2), © Erica Guilane-Nachez, Fotolia, (3), © Charlotte Frearson

Figure 11.1: page 149, © Helen Hotson, Fotolia

Page 151, © Iriana Papoyan, Fotolia

Page 153, © ArenaCreative, Fotolia

Page 156, © Alexey Fedorenko, Fotolia

Figure 12.1: page 160, © Morphart, Fotolia

Figure 12.2: page 164, © Erica Guilane-Nachez, Fotolia

Figure 12.3: page 169 © acrogame, Fotolia

Figure 13.1: page 174, © Charlotte Frearson

Figure 13.2: page 176, © Erica Guilane-Nachez, Fotolia

Figure 14.1: page 187, © Tanya, Fotolia

Page 192, © Charlotte Frearson

Figure 15.1: page 205, © Erica Guilane-Nachez, Fotolia

Page 210, © Erica Guilane-Nachez, Fotolia

Page 211, © Erica Guilane-Nachez, Fotolia

Page 212, © Erica Guilane-Nachez, Fotolia

Page 213, © RetroClipArt, Fotolia

Page 214, © ag visuell, Fotolia

Appendix 1: page 225, © Erica Guilane-Nachez, Fotolia

Appendix 2: page 229, © Erica Guilane-Nachez, Fotolia

Appendix 3: page 233, © Tony Baggett, Fotolia

Appendix 4: page 237, © acrogame, Fotolia